Invisible
ADHD

Invisible ADHD

Proven Mood and Life Management for Smart yet Scattered Women

Shanna Pearson

Founder and President, Expert ADHD Coaching
ADHDcoaching.com
Transforming Lives for Adults with ADHD Since 1999

Foreword by Daniel G. Amen, MD

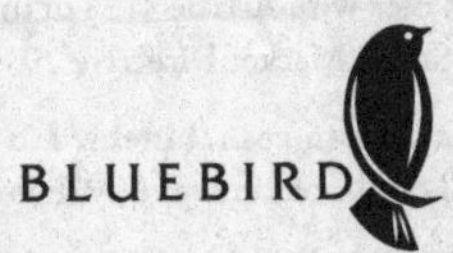

First published 2025 by Flatiron Books

First published in the UK 2025 by Bluebird
an imprint of Pan Macmillan
The Smithson, 6 Briset Street, London EC1M 5NR
EU representative: Macmillan Publishers Ireland Ltd, 1st Floor,
The Liffey Trust Centre, 117–126 Sheriff Street Upper,
Dublin 1 D01 YC43
Associated companies throughout the world

ISBN 978-1-0350-8266-7

Copyright © Shanna Pearson 2025
Foreword copyright © Daniel G. Amen 2025

Author's Note: The information in this book, by necessity, is of a general nature and should not be considered a substitute for an individual evaluation or treatment by the reader's own physician or other competent medical professional. Individual readers are solely responsible for their own health care decisions. You should always consult a medical professional on matters relating to your health, especially if you have existing medical conditions, and before starting, stopping, or changing any existing health regimen or the dose of any medication you are taking. If you believe you are in need of medical intervention, please see a medical practitioner as soon as possible. The author and publisher do not accept responsibility for any adverse effects individuals may claim to experience, whether directly or indirectly, from the information contained in this book. Finally, although the case studies in this book are real, the names and circumstances of those profiled have been changed to protect client/patient anonymity.

The right of Shanna Pearson to be identified as the author of this work has been asserted in accordance with the Copyright, Designs and Patents Act 1988.

All rights reserved. No part of this publication may be reproduced, stored in a retrieval system, or transmitted, in any form, or by any means (including, without limitation, electronic, mechanical, photocopying, recording or otherwise) without the prior written permission of the publisher.

Pan Macmillan does not have any control over, or any responsibility for, any author or third-party websites (including, without limitation, URLs, emails and QR codes) referred to in or on this book.

2

A CIP catalogue record for this book is available from the British Library.

Printed and bound in India at Repro India Ltd., Mumbai

This book is sold subject to the condition that it shall not, by way of trade or otherwise, be lent, hired out, or otherwise circulated without the publisher's prior consent in any form of binding or cover other than that in which it is published and without a similar condition including this condition being imposed on the subsequent purchaser. The publisher does not authorize the use or reproduction of any part of this book in any manner for the purpose of training artificial intelligence technologies or systems. The publisher expressly reserves this book from the Text and Data Mining exception in accordance with Article 4(3) of the European Union Digital Single Market Directive 2019/790.

Visit **www.panmacmillan.com/bluebird** to read more about all our books and to buy them.

For sale in the Indian subcontinent only

To Jeremy: for every. single. thing.

—and to Arielle and Izach, my favorite reasons
I still get to live what's in this book every day.

—and to my parents, for never actually selling me
to the highest (or was it lowest?) bidder.

With so much love.

Contents

Foreword

When it comes to ADHD, few people have seen and studied it as closely as I have. At Amen Clinics, we've diagnosed and treated tens of thousands of individuals with ADHD—likely more than any other medical or psychiatric clinic in the world. In 1991, I started using sophisticated brain-imaging techniques to understand how we can help people better by looking at the physical functioning of their brains in conjunction with their symptoms. The brain scans made it clear to me that taking care of the physical health of the brain improves cognition and conditions like ADHD as well. Therefore, by focusing on brain health alongside symptoms, we've helped people improve cognitive function and overall quality of life.

But brain health alone isn't the whole story. Adults with ADHD also need something just as vital: practical behavioral strategies, skills, an empowered mindset, and daily habits that support long-term growth and change. This is where Shanna Pearson comes in.

Shanna is the founder of Expert ADHD Coaching, and I'm a big fan. My team of doctors has referred patients to her coaching program because we know that the "nonmedical" side of ADHD management is just as essential as the clinical side. Shanna's unique insight and coaching program addresses a critical gap—the place where daily actions and habits intersect with mental well-being. This type of coaching gives people the tools and deeper understanding to create and stick with new habits, increase their self-confidence, manage their time and their ever-changing moods, and feel more in control of their lives. And while the type of behavioral therapy she provides certainly requires specialized approaches and experience, what sets Shanna apart is her extraordinary insight and remarkable instinct for exactly what each person needs to do in their individual situations.

This is why I'm happy to introduce this book to you. Shanna's incredible "action-first" approach is not just a concept—it's a proven method! Her work with people with ADHD focuses on small, practical, and consistent changes that produce lasting results. The stories we have heard from our patients about their experiences with her program are inspiring. These aren't just stories of survival—they're stories of breakthroughs, where people finally feel like they're in control of their lives for the first time.

If you've ever wanted a behind-the-scenes look at the inner world of women with ADHD, this book delivers. Shanna goes far beneath the surface to explore the "why" behind the everyday struggles women with ADHD face. But she doesn't stop there.

She's been in the trenches, listening, guiding, and coaching women through their journeys. She's taken that experience, as well as her own personal journey living with ADHD, and turned it into a clear, powerful guide for anyone with ADHD who's felt invisible, misunderstood, or overwhelmed. This book offers more than insight—it offers solutions.

Here's what's different about Shanna's approach: She's not here to talk about theory. She's here to help you understand what you actually need to do in your life to work with your ADHD instead of against it. Her book provides incredible insight and practical guidance—tools, techniques, and strategies that she has developed to help people with ADHD shift from feeling stuck to becoming unstoppable. You'll learn how to regulate your emotions, follow through and get things done, manage your overwhelm, build your self-worth, and finally feel like you're on top of life in a way that works for YOU.

In the world of ADHD behavior management, I've seen very few people as insightful and capable as Shanna Pearson. Her expertise is undeniable, her compassion is genuine, and her incredible track record of results speaks for itself.

If you're ready to understand the "why" behind many of the struggles that come with ADHD and, more importantly, the "how" to move forward with confidence, this book is for you, and I encourage you to take this opportunity to learn from one of the best.

Daniel G. Amen, MD
Founder, Amen Clinics

Invisible
ADHD

Proven Mood and Life Management
for Smart yet Scattered Women

Introduction

"Why Can't You Just . . .?"

I can still remember a night in May when I was six years old. I was about to finish first grade and was counting down the days until school let out for summer, when our family dinner was interrupted by a phone call from my teacher.

According to her records, I had not turned in my homework. Not just that day; I hadn't turned in any homework since *November*. As a result, they were considering holding me back a year.

Not only was this news to my parents, it was also news to me. Homework? When had the teacher given us homework? I couldn't remember. My parents were furious—not with me but with the teacher. Why, they demanded, had she waited the entire year to let them know about this? And how was this my fault?

Nobody ever asked *me* why I hadn't turned in my homework. Or why I never knew that we had any. Nobody spent time observing or really noticing me in class—I was essentially invisible. No one ever knew what was really going on with me. Not my teachers. Not my parents. Not even me.

At school, I was always the spacey daydreamer. I stared out the window for unknown periods of time. I gave random answers to questions. A teacher would give directions, but I wouldn't realize it until I saw everyone pulling out books or scribbling on their papers. I watched my classmates for clues. "Wait . . . *what* do we have to do?"

While I never got my teachers' instructions the first time, I *definitely* got their exasperation. I became very familiar with the phrase *Why can't you just . . . ?* As in:

"*Why can't you just* pay attention?"
"*Why can't you just* follow directions?"
"*Why can't you just* finish your homework?"

I never knew what was going on in class and was terrified of being called on, so I learned to keep a low profile at school. But at home, that was impossible. I was a perpetual non-finisher of chores, activities, meals, and conversations. The same refrain I heard at school became an ongoing theme at home, too.

"*Why can't you just* eat your dinner?"
"*Why can't you just* stop interrupting?"
"*Why can't you just* do what you said you were going to do?"

Nobody had any idea how badly I wanted to meet people's expectations. Nobody saw how the thing I'd just started was so much more interesting than the thing I hadn't finished yet. It felt like there was something about me that would always be misunderstood, which had me believe there was something fundamentally wrong with me, and I had no idea what it was.

Nobody knew it then, and actually wouldn't for many years, but the root of all these problems was undiagnosed ADHD. Perhaps you can relate?

A SECRET SORORITY

Most people associate ADHD with hyperactivity, but for many women, a lot of our "hyperactivity" is internal and therefore totally *invisible*. It likely wasn't evident to your teachers when you were younger. Instead, the boys with ADHD, who were usually much more physically disruptive and loud (especially with bodily function noises), were noticed and called out more. Their parents received the most teacher phone calls and may have been advised to seek help from their child's pediatrician.

So *of course* these hyperactive kids got a ton of attention—they were driving their parents, teachers, and most of the other kids in class nuts!

But that wasn't you. Nope. Even in high school, it was more likely that you were the quiet, incessant daydreamer, distracted by the 24–7 amusement park in your brain and managed to fly completely under the radar. You were focusing on your real and imagined life, including radical (yet absolutely brilliant!) ideas, creating complicated dramas in your mind, imagining winning very important life-altering arguments, living your "best" life looking gorgeous at a raging party with your two hundred best friends, accepting a major and meaningful award while your ex (the one who broke your heart) is watching longingly from the audience, or wondering what your dog dreams about.

But now, you wake up one day in your thirties, forties, or sixties wondering why (whhyyy?!?) your life is twenty times more stressful than everyone else's and why everyone you know seems to have their act together while you're still living in total chaos looking for the cup of coffee you were holding just a minute ago. You may feel as if you have been trying to head in a particular direction and have goals or dreams you want to fulfill but are always getting sidetracked and taken way off course. If you have achieved career success, you may feel like you're only a step away from being called out as a fraud or getting fired; either that or you're running around at ninety miles an hour, nonstop, feeling like you're still not even remotely close to getting what you really want.

Why *does* it seem that your life has always been much more tumultuous than most? Why *is* it more of a struggle to achieve anything meaningful to you? Why has it *always* felt that no one really gets you? Why *do* you seem to exist on a completely different frequency from everyone else around you?

The answer, and a big lesson from this book, is that your brain functions differently from a lot of people's, *and* there is nothing wrong with you. You're going to learn how your brain works (or in your case, works differently) and that there are even a few gifts associated with ADHD. You'll learn how to recognize the ADHD characteristics that are most likely getting in your way and discover new ways of thinking about and doing things that work *with* your brain and not against it. In addition to a few of my own personal experiences, you'll also read about other women who struggled with aspects of their ADHD and have learned to overcome them. These are 100 percent true experiences of real women from my ADHD coaching company, Expert ADHD Coaching.

WHY SHOULD YOU LISTEN TO ME?

You may have already read other books on ADHD, followed ADHD influencers, or watched countless life hacks online, and chances are you've gathered a ton of information, but how much of a difference has it truly made in your life? I'll guess probably a little bit, but maybe not as much as you'd hoped. Which brings me to what's different about this book and why you should listen to me.

First, if you're a woman with ADHD, I honestly get what you are struggling with. I've been there—and am still there! I know exactly what it feels like, and I have solutions to share with you that can help make your life much easier.

Second, and *much* more importantly, my coaching practice has grown to be the world's largest one-on-one coaching company specifically for adults with ADHD, and the solutions I'll be sharing with you are based on twenty-six years of **proven results** with tens of thousands of clients!

I am truly humbled and amazed that since 1999 I have had the privilege to coach and manage more than four hundred and fifty thousand (450,000) individual ADHD coaching sessions, and we now conduct almost *sixty thousand* one-hour coaching sessions every single year. I have personally trained hundreds of ADHD coaches, many of whom still work for my company and continue to be under my guidance every day, and prominent physicians and psychiatrists across North America regularly refer their patients to my program.

To be clear, these are *not* social media followers, online group members, or podcast listeners seeking free information (honestly, I'm not very active on social media since most clients find us through referrals). Almost anyone can accumulate thousands of unpaid subscribers in a large free group and then claim they have "coached" and "helped" thousands of people, often without offering proven advice. My numbers are based on the results of thousands of paying clients who are guided over time, individually, *one-on-one,* through their unique and specific challenges. Even with all the free information available, our clients invest a substantial amount for my concierge, results-based adult ADHD program because *what we do really works.*

One of the reasons I wrote this book is to give access to the information, experience, and insight I have developed over the years to as many people as possible, not just those who can participate in our program.

Finally, I promise to tell you the truth, and I'm not going to sugarcoat anything. I'm not going to give you "theoretical" solutions that look interesting and sound good but haven't really been tested in real life, and I'm *not* going to tell you that ADHD is a magical "superpower" when you know all too well how hard it is to just be you.

Everything I'm going to share with you reflects my experience and the extraordinary results I've seen with my clients over many years. All the techniques and strategies presented here have been proven to work for literally thousands of women with ADHD, some of whom are probably a lot like you!

IMPLEMENTATION IS THE ONLY WAY TO ACHIEVE REAL RESULTS!

Most of us think we already know something if we've read or heard it before, but that's just learning and knowing *about* something. We all have access to the internet on our phones, and we can look up anything about everything—anytime we want! So, when it comes to new tools or practices that will help you in your life, it's only when you actually *use* them in your life that you'll *really* know them.

At this point, after working with all our clients throughout the years, we've learned what gets results, as well as what doesn't—even if it's portrayed on social media and elsewhere as *the* thing *everyone* is doing.

"Action-First" Behavior Modification Training

The foundation of my entire ADHD coaching program is the exact opposite of many popular philosophies that focus on changing our thoughts and beliefs first, which is incredibly difficult when you have an overflowing, everything-all-at-once, high-speed brain. My philosophy is based on highly *directive* kinesthetic learning, which is more akin to athletic coaching than typical ADHD life coaching. Basically, your actions will create your results, and your results, in turn, will reshape your thoughts and beliefs about yourself.

Just as I do with all my clients, I'll be guiding you throughout this book to take specific actions and do things in a specific way that will lead to remarkable results. So, when (not if) you read about something here that makes you roll your eyes because you think it's too simple or obvious, or annoying, or is too "out there" or "I already know that," please don't dismiss it. Every client we've ever had has argued with their coach at some point about why something we ask them to try definitely won't work, or won't make a difference, or is way too basic for them—until they actually do it every day for a week, and then they (usually) change their tune.

The information and techniques I'll be sharing in these pages have been changing lives for decades, and the only way you'll ever know what works, especially what will work for YOU, is when you incorporate it into your actual day-to-day life. If you practice just a few of the tips you learn in this book, I'm convinced your life will become much easier and more fulfilling. I believe that deeply. After all, that's why I wrote this book for you.

What You'll Discover

You'll uncover a new understanding of ADHD and gain much deeper insight into yourself, all while gaining countless strategies that not only simplify your daily life but help you thrive in ways you never thought possible.

Here's how we'll progress:

- **Part 1: The WHAT**—A short and sweet overview of ADHD essentials.
- **Part 2: The WHY**—Insight into the source of many of your persistent personality "quirks," your ever-changing emotions, and why you do the things you do that don't ever work for you.
- **Part 3: The TOOLS**—Easy and proven strategies, exercises, and tools that will ensure you manage your ADHD effectively in a way that works for you and your life.
- **Part 4: What's NEXT**—Strengthening your confidence, self-esteem, and self-trust, to bring your unique brilliance and awesomeness to the world!

What You'll Need

Besides an open mind, I suggest having a notebook with you to use frequently as you go through this book. It will be a place to do the exercises, record your answers and responses, and keep track of what you learn and the skills you are acquiring. As you'll discover, it can be very helpful to write down information rather than just adding yet one more thought onto an already overflowing pile of ideas you won't remember later. Also, when you physically write things down, rather than typing on a keyboard or on your phone, it forces your brain to slow down and you can retain that information better.

So, in case you forget, go get a notebook and pen now. I'll wait for you here.

What You'll Do

In addition to uncovering brand-new insights about yourself throughout this book, Parts 3 and 4 provide powerful techniques and strategies for you to apply in your own life! These will be marked with this "For-YOU-To-Do" icon: ☑.

At the end of each chapter in part 3, you'll find the One Focus exercise—a signature process of our coaching program. By practicing one small habit-changing technique or behavior every day for a week, you can begin to reinforce a concept that you learn in each chapter until it becomes something that you can incorporate into your life *for good.* You can write down your One Focus in your notebook, or post it where you'll see it every day, so that you'll remember to do it all week.

What You'll Get

I promise you are going to read some things here that you won't find in your average get-organized, manage-your-time-better-for-people-with-ADHD book. You are going to learn the counterpoint to what most people say (and you may have come to believe) about ADHD and learn how people with ADHD (yes, including you) can absolutely focus, pay attention, manage their emotions, be productive, be organized, and follow through on just about anything!

You'll understand that you are not broken. You are not your ADHD. You have just been trying to work inside a system that wasn't built for your brain. You'll get all this and much more. So let's get started!

PART I

Your Brain on ADHD

1

Your Brain Isn't Broken, Just Different!

You may have already been diagnosed with ADHD, or you may *think* you have ADHD, but in either case, you have likely been dealing with overwhelm, distraction, discontent, inner restlessness, procrastination, forgetfulness, impulsivity, and more for some time now. Although you know you're a pretty quick thinker—and maybe even smarter than most—you may also feel frustrated, internally restless, and unable to achieve what you most want in your life. You may have wondered, *Why can't I do things like everyone else?* or *What the #!*%! is wrong with me?* You may have spent a lifetime asking yourself these questions and possibly didn't suspect you had ADHD until you were an adult. For most of your life, you may have heard family, friends, teachers, and bosses (basically, the more important people in your world) exclaim, "Why can't you *just* . . . !?" You heard this line so often that it became a chorus installed on repeat, now living rent-free in your head! Well, the reason you "can't just . . ." is that your brain works a bit differently from a "neurotypical" brain (whatever "typical" means).

There are a lot of different theories about ADHD, and you can go down a deep rabbit hole on the internet looking into it if you'd like, but the first thing to know about ADHD is that it is *real*. If you have it, you were born with it. You don't get it from eating sugary cereal loaded with red dye, cell phone radiation, childhood trauma, or having too much screen time as a kid. Yes, screen time, radiation, food additives, trauma, and *many* other factors can contribute to exacerbating, and mimicking, ADHD symptoms;

however, they are not the *cause* of ADHD. The symptoms we associate with ADHD occur because of how our brains are wired.

Just like you don't need to know how an internal combustion engine operates to drive a car, you don't need to know all the scientific ins and outs to get insight into your ADHD. Many of our clients, especially those who are doctors, already know a tremendous amount about the human brain, but that knowledge hasn't ever helped them make changes in their everyday lives. Which is why this isn't a book about science or the biochemistry of the ADHD brain. That said, knowing a few key bits of information can help you better understand why you think the way you think, feel the way you feel, and do things the way you do them. So here are some basics.

KEY POINT #1: ADHD is real (I know I said it before, but it bears repeating), and it's a lifelong condition that can affect anyone. It's also highly genetic, so you can blame your parents! (Not really. Well, okay, maybe a bit.) So, if you have ADHD, or think you might, there is a strong possibility that someone closely related to you has it, too.

KEY POINT #2: ADHD is a disorder of *regulating attention and emotion,* and the challenges associated with it are due to biochemical differences in how your brain functions. Organization, information processing, focus, as well as impulse control, self-soothing, and moderating difficult emotions are very challenging for adults with ADHD.

KEY POINT #3: You are not your brain. Well, maybe you are; it's debatable. That said, it's certain that you are definitely *not* your ADHD. You are so much more! Understanding a bit about your brain will allow you to use its incredible power to become more of who you want to be with the freedom to accomplish what's most important to you.

I'm going to dig a little deeper for a minute into how the ADHD brain works. Feel free to stick around for some nontechnical science or, if you'd rather not, skip ahead a few pages to where it says, "*Official End to Brain Science Info*" and I'll meet you there!

ADHD AND YOUR BRAIN

There are a lot of theories about ADHD, and no one is 100 percent certain how and why it occurs. It is still the subject of ongoing research, and over the past few decades, there have been several ways of describing and identifying it. Although conditions similar to what we now call ADHD have been described since 1798, ADHD was only first recognized diagnostically by the American Psychiatric Association in the 1968 publication of the *Diagnostic and Statistical Manual of Mental Disorders*, second edition (*DSM-II*). At the time, it was thought to be a condition of young children—primarily boys—and was initially called "Hyperkinetic Reaction of Childhood." The perception has evolved from being a disorder of excessive motor activity to that of attention deficit (with and without hyperactivity) and now is known as ADHD with three main subtypes.[1]

1. **ADHD—predominantly hyperactive impulsive:** This type is much more noticeable and disruptive to others because it shows up physically. Behaviors can easily be seen and heard, such as difficulty sitting still, constant fidgeting, talking nonstop, being loud and disruptive, interrupting, calling out of turn, and being physically restless and often in motion.

2. **ADHD-I—predominantly inattentive:** This is a much quieter form of ADHD, as the hyperactive component exists almost entirely internally. Someone with ADHD-I can be extremely forgetful and have trouble listening and following directions. They can get totally lost in their thoughts, often daydreaming, worrying, ruminating, being indecisive, and overanalyzing absolutely everything. They can become consumed for hours

in their own ever-changing and entertaining ideas and totally lose contact with what is happening around them.

3. **ADHD-COMBINED—symptoms of both inattention and hyperactivity-impulsivity:** With this form of ADHD, the person can have hyperactivity and inattention; impulsiveness and distractibility.

It was originally thought that kids "outgrew" their ADHD, and it's only recently that ADHD was recognized as a problem that persists into and throughout adulthood. There's also been a closer look at ADHD in different populations, and most recently in different genders—it generally shows up as inattention in women and visible hyperactivity in men. The word *generally* can't be overstated here, as there are *plenty* of women (including me) who also have the visibly hyperactive component.

Thankfully, we now have a consensus that ADHD is caused by differences in brain biochemistry. Here's how that works:

***Norepinephrine / Dopamine Uptake*:** Norepinephrine is a neurotransmitter that is connected to stress and the fight-or-flight response. Dopamine is another neurotransmitter that is linked to motivation, the ability to take action in order to achieve specific results, emotional regulation, and more. When you have ADHD, your brain doesn't use these neurotransmitters as effectively as it could, either because you are producing less of the neurotransmitter, resulting in a deficiency, or because the neurotransmitters are available but the receptors for them are blocked so less of the neurotransmitter enters your brain. When you have ADHD, these lower levels of norepinephrine and dopamine affect various regions of your brain that govern the way you behave. Let's take a closer look:

***Limbic System*:** The limbic system is located deep in the middle of your brain with the primary job of regulating your emotions and your behaviors. It is one of the oldest and most primitive brain structures, dating back to the early evolution of mammals. It plays a big role in your fight-or-flight responses, your memory, and attaching emotional content to your memories. So you can imagine the results when there's a lag in this brain region. When the emotional part of the brain is unregulated, you can experience low frustration tolerance, heightened aggression, impatience, and raw or unmoderated emotions.

***Basal Ganglia*:** The basal ganglia comprise a group of nuclei located deep within your brain that play a role in cognition, motivation behavior, and emotional processing. It's like Grand Central Station, where neural circuits serve as the control center for all information entering your brain and send the information to the exact locations in your brain that need it. Issues here can cause the information entering the brain to be misdirected, so you can have that panicky lost feeling of "What the heck am I supposed to do?" or being pulled in different directions by disjointed emotions. Any challenges or deficiencies in this region can result in inattention, distractibility, or impulsivity.

***Prefrontal Cortex*:** Located right behind your forehead, the prefrontal cortex is responsible for executive function and cognitive skills like prioritization, holding attention, and organizational skills. One of its main jobs is to act as a filter or gatekeeper. It assesses the significance of situations, calculates the costs of your reactions, and ideally holds your impulsive actions at bay. When there are issues in this area and your gatekeeper is "off duty," it is very difficult to filter and prioritize what's coming into your brain. All information, worries, and decisions seem to have the exact same level of importance and are all lumped together in one big holding area instead of being filed away in nicely organized compartments, and every waking moment of your life can feel like "everything all at once right now!"

Official End to Brain Science Info

My point in talking about this is to emphasize that your brain is wired differently in a way that contributes to you being the amazing, dynamic, creative, yet potentially stressed-out, frustrated, and overwhelmed person you are. But that's not all. In my experience, there are three specific fundamental challenges that most women with ADHD share, yet often don't understand or aren't even aware of. So let's look at these next.

2

The Three Most Important Things That You and Everyone Who Knows You Must Understand About ADHD

After more than twenty years of speaking one-on-one with thousands of women with ADHD across all ages, cultures, countries, economic situations, careers, and so on, I've found that three core characteristics are the source of our most problematic ADHD behaviors. Once you and everyone who cares about you understand what these "Big Three" are, your behaviors will (finally!) make sense!

#1: Our Unconscious Need to Create Stimulus

When your brain doesn't receive enough stimulation due to a deficiency of neurotransmitters, it looks for a workaround, manufacturing that stimulation in other ways. In addition to ADHD medications, the majority of which are stimulants, many of us unconsciously seek out and create stimuli in our everyday moments and naturally gravitate toward what feels the most captivating—even if we know it's not in our best interest.

Many of us unconsciously seek out and create stimuli in our everyday moments.

Maybe you have found yourself waiting until the last minute, jumping from one thing to the next and not following through on anything, or being oppositional or argumentative with people especially (ironically) when things get "too" comfortable. Perhaps you become fully immersed in "feels interesting right now" distractions like social media, or unconsciously creating drama and upheaval in your career, your family, your relationships, or anything else you can name! It's all part of your incredible brain's attempt to keep itself engaged. The problem is that a lot of the stimulus you seek ends up working *against* you and gets in the way of achieving what you want. We'll be getting into this in much more detail in part 2, and you may be surprised to find that some of your more notable character traits and behaviors come directly from this need!

#2: Difficulty Compartmentalizing

Your incredible brain has a very difficult time focusing on one thing at a time, or keeping one thought separate from another. Imagine that a thought about a situation can be squished up and tightly contained into a space the size of a golf ball. That's how most neurotypical people would handle a thought. For us ADHDers, it's very different because the thought cannot be contained. In fact, that same thought is more like a liquid without a container, and it spills and leaks and becomes absorbed by everything around it. Even when you believe your thoughts or emotions are somewhat contained, in the middle of a random moment, you notice them slowly seeping into whatever you are doing and thinking about, demanding you pay attention to them immediately before they cause collateral damage! When there's no containment for your thoughts and emotions, everything seems and feels all-encompassing, all the time. I call this "the ADHD Brain's Inability to Compartmentalize," and it impacts almost everything you do! It's never *just* about not being able to prioritize your thoughts or to-do list or getting that project done on time. Your all-encompassing "everything all at once right now" reality impacts your relationship with time, with life, with others, and most importantly, with yourself.

When there's no containment for your thoughts and emotions, everything seems and feels all-encompassing, all the time. I call this "the ADHD Brain's Inability to Compartmentalize," and it impacts almost everything you do.

#3: Flooded by Overwhelm

One major outcome of having a brain that has difficulty compartmentalizing is overwhelm. It's such a common challenge that "Overwhelmed All the Time" could be the official tagline for ADHD because so many of our ADHD traits and behaviors can be traced back to being overwhelmed or trying to escape the clutches of overwhelm!

The experience of having so many things going on in your mind at the same time can make you feel metaphorically paralyzed. Every thought in your head takes up the exact same amount of space with equal importance and becomes one gigantic thing whirled together, impossible to separate, until you become flooded. Flooded with feelings, flooded with thoughts, and flooded with possibilities, which could describe the inner experience of almost every woman with ADHD.

"Overwhelmed All the Time" could be the official tagline for ADHD.

This state of overwhelm makes it difficult to start things, move forward, be present with others, or even think straight, and is often the underlying source of our most common ADHD symptoms like procrastination, disorganization, distraction, impulsivity, time blindness, and indecision.

WHAT WORKS FOR OTHERS WON'T WORK FOR YOU

I've had so many people tell me that they legitimately think there's something "wrong" with them because they've been trying to manage their time, be more productive, get organized, and be less overwhelmed in the same way that their friends and most neurotypical people do, and it hasn't worked! But insisting on doing things the exact same way everyone else does when you are *not* wired like everyone else will leave you frustrated and annoyed for the rest of your life! And you deserve much better.

Think of it this way: Most people who have very curly hair know they need to use a different brush (or not use one at all), hair cleansers, conditioners, and styling products (even pillowcases!) than their straight-haired friends do. They're not "broken" or "wrong" for having curly hair, and except for the extra hair-care time, it is really not a major concern. Even if they once found their hair impossible to deal with, once they know what to do differently, it gets easier and looks amazing!

Insisting on doing things the exact same way everyone else does when you are *not* wired like everyone else will leave you frustrated and annoyed for the rest of your life! And you deserve much better.

Trying to manage your ADHD symptoms with the same tools that are suited to someone who is neurotypical just won't work. You *know* you need to send that email, write that paper, pay those bills, feel and show gratitude for the good things in your life, stop working by 5:30 p.m. to be on time for dinner, do your laundry, eat more protein and less sugar, get out of bed when the alarm rings, or leave for work on time. And although these things seem simple (we all know *how* to get out of bed!), you need to go from *knowing* what to do to actually *doing* things differently. In this book, you'll learn how to take action on the things you most want to do in a way that *works* for your amazing ADHD brain. But before we get to that, let's clarify one important thing. Because society as a whole has become so unbelievably loud with nonstop stimuli and distractions, it makes it nearly impossible for *anyone* to be totally present and focused. So how do you even know, for sure, if you actually have ADHD?

3

Is It Really ADHD?

Getting a Diagnosis

In my early thirties, I ended up in a situation that traumatized me for years. My life had suddenly flipped upside down and fallen apart so disastrously that it was unrecognizable. At one point I had to temporarily move back home with my parents because I had nowhere else to go—so I wasn't exactly feeling my "best." When I was visiting with a friend, his dad (who happened to be a psychiatrist) overheard me talking about what was going on in my life and how I was feeling about it. He straight out asked if I had been diagnosed with ADHD. I thought that was a bit odd because at the time I thought only kids had ADHD.

He got me an appointment with a colleague, who administered a self-assessment questionnaire and, based on how I responded that day, diagnosed me with depression. This didn't make sense to me, because although my life seemed incredibly depressing at that moment, it wasn't always like that. I honestly didn't feel depressed. She then prescribed an antidepressant, which actually did *make me feel depressed, so I stopped taking it almost immediately.*

I asked my friend's dad if there was another option, and this time, he sent me to an ADHD specialist. This doctor didn't just want to know how I was feeling at the time; he wanted to dig into my entire life, and asked me to bring my childhood report cards to the assessment. Luckily, my mom still had them—all the way back to kindergarten (wow, go Mom!). I never realized this while growing up, but every year from kindergarten to high school, my teachers wrote comments about my not paying attention, talking out of turn, being forgetful, "daydreaming the days away," and only tuning in if I knew there was an upcoming test. The doctor gave me not one but three different diagnostic tests, talked to me about my past jobs and relationships, and essentially investigated how I had lived throughout my entire life. He was looking at the movie and not just a snapshot, and eventually, he diagnosed me with severe ADHD. He actually told me that I was the "poster child for extreme ADHD."

Everything Made Sense

As soon as he said it, I almost wanted to cry from relief. I literally got goose bumps over my whole body—it felt so true. Everything, I mean everything, in my life, my work, my need to always be in motion, going from relationship to relationship, place to place, idea to idea, now, finally, all made sense! And now that I knew what was going on, I could hopefully figure out how to fix it!

Just about every person on the planet feels overwhelmed, inattentive, impulsive, unproductive, disorganized, restless, or exhibits other common ADHD traits at some point, but that doesn't mean that they have ADHD. If you've exhibited symptoms or behaviors of ADHD consistently throughout your *entire life*, and not just in the past few years in response to major life stressors or external events when life feels distracting for everyone, then it's possible that you're dealing with ADHD.

Some of the challenges in identifying ADHD are similar to other mental health differences and lie in the fact that there is no widely used physical test, blood test, X-ray, or MRI that can definitively diagnose ADHD. The only way to know if you have it is through undergoing a detailed evaluation, which is typically done by a health care provider. Because the testing is generally based on psychological self-evaluation, and the answers to the questions can depend on how you happen to be feeling on that particular day, a definitive diagnosis can sometimes be difficult! Additionally, some doctors use qEEG brain mapping or brain SPECT scans to identify ADHD; however, there still isn't a consensus in the medical community on their use as a diagnostic tool.

To make things even murkier, ADHD varies from person to person, and your exact ADHD symptoms aren't going to be the same as your best friend's or your ex's. For example, some people with ADHD are extremely successful in their careers, but their personal lives are a disaster. Or they are super organized at home and able to stay on top of everything for their family members, but at their job, they're all over the place. Some of us may be unable to focus unless simultaneously listening to music while others need complete silence to concentrate. Some are excessively emotional; others have a hard time feeling and connecting to their emotions at all. Ultimately, those with ADHD exhibit a range of traits that are connected to self-regulation of attention, actions, and emotions.

It's also important to know that just because you were not diagnosed with ADHD as a kid doesn't mean you don't have ADHD. Because the most common and difficult symptoms for women are often emotional, women who suffer from ADHD-related mood dysregulation were (and still are) frequently dismissed with "She's just overly emotional" or "It must be that time of the month" instead of getting a proper evaluation or being taken seriously. This leads to many women with ADHD living their *entire lives* undiagnosed or being misdiagnosed with something else entirely!

MISDIAGNOSIS: ANXIETY AND DEPRESSION

Sometimes the symptoms of ADHD can overlap with the symptoms of other mood disorders. For many women, living with symptoms like emotional dysregulation, impulsivity, lack of confidence, and social challenges often can contribute to feelings of low self-worth and anxiety. Low self-esteem, occasional feelings of hopelessness, and oversensitivity related to ADHD can look like depression, even if you are not truly depressed! For those reasons, and because a woman with ADHD is more likely to be a daydreamer than a disrupter, many of us have been misdiagnosed with depression and anxiety. To complicate things further, many women actually *do* have comorbid anxiety, depression, or other conditions alongside their ADHD and live their entire lives never having the full picture of what is going on with them. Additionally, if you're misdiagnosed then the medication you're prescribed won't help the way it should and you can feel even more discouraged and think that you will never find a solution for your situation. Once you know that you have ADHD, you can receive proper treatment, and everything can be managed simultaneously.

Women who suffer from ADHD-related mood dysregulation were (and still are) frequently dismissed with "She's just overly emotional" or "It must be that time of the month" instead of getting a proper evaluation or being taken seriously. This leads to many women with ADHD living their *entire* lives undiagnosed or being misdiagnosed with something else entirely!

GETTING A CORRECT DIAGNOSIS AND FINDING A PRACTITIONER WHO GETS IT—AND YOU

It is important that you find a professional psychologist, psychiatrist, or physician who specializes in ADHD. A doctor will diagnose ADHD using the criteria in the *DSM* (the official manual of psychiatric conditions in the United States), which lists nine symptoms that suggest inattentive, and another nine symptoms for hyperactive/impulsive. You need to have five or six specific symptoms consistently throughout your life, and in different settings, for a diagnosis to be made.

Remember, there is not one single test or evaluation that will determine whether you definitively have ADHD. It can take a lot of digging into past school and other performance to get to a diagnosis. Even academic performance can sometimes be misleading. I know a college student who was discussing ADHD with her psychiatrist, and the psychiatrist asked about her grades. Her grades were excellent, so the doctor told her she probably doesn't have ADHD. What he didn't ask about was how much extra time, colossal effort, and all-nighters it took to overcome her disorganization and distraction to get those good grades. Subsequently, she worked with another psychiatrist, who went much deeper and properly diagnosed her with ADHD-I. Now, with a combination of medication, new skills, and strategies, she is able to get the same academic results without having to work so frustratingly long and hard.

Although it may be tempting (and quicker) to self-diagnose with online quizzes, the only thing that you can really learn from these is whether it might make sense to pursue an actual professional medical evaluation, which can take many hours. It may seem like a lot to go through, but for many women, being diagnosed with ADHD as an adult is an incredibly validating and empowering experience that brings a massive feeling of relief and realization of "finally my entire life makes sense!"

Regardless of what stage of life you're in, whether you're seventeen or eighty-seven years old, a correct diagnosis can be liberating, empowering, and, with the right help, completely life-changing.

But soon, you may wonder what's next. What are you supposed to do now? It's possible that the doctor who diagnosed you will also write you a prescription for ADHD medication, but just because you have a prescription in hand doesn't mean all your problems are solved. This is only the beginning!

4

ADHD Medication and Management

Pills Don't Teach Skills

When used properly, medication can be an *extremely* helpful and sometimes necessary step to treating ADHD, but it won't ever *fix* your ADHD, make it go away, or give you effective ways to manage your ADHD (at least not unless your prescription comes with a personal assistant). I've had many coaching clients over the years describe their medication as a lifesaving oxygen mask! Conversely, I've also had clients say they feel worse and have a hard time functioning when taking their ADHD medication.

Either way, medication *alone* usually isn't the answer, but unfortunately, most newly diagnosed women get a prescription and nothing else. Many of our clients come to me after taking ADHD medication for years—decades even—yet they're still desperately looking for help because they never learned the skills they need to move forward in their lives.

One of the benefits of ADHD medication is that it can really help you stay focused; *however,* it doesn't help you stay focused on the "right" things. Which means you can take your medication and stay extremely focused on your social media feed for five hours straight (not that you would ever do that) when it only feels like twenty minutes.

Many of our clients come to me after taking ADHD medication for years—decades, even—yet they're still desperately looking for help because they never learned the skills they need to move forward in their lives.

This helps explain why numerous studies show that the most effective treatment plan to manage ADHD is a multimodal approach combining medication with behavioral treatment to learn *how* to do things differently.

MEDICATIONS FOR ADHD

ADHD medications fall into two groups—stimulants and non-stimulants.

Stimulants

As you now know, your brain seeks out stimulus to compensate for lower dopamine and norepinephrine levels, so it's no surprise that many ADHD medications are stimulant based to help people gain focus, be more attentive, reduce distractibility, and aid in impulse and emotional control. It may seem a bit counterintuitive to give someone who can be physically or emotionally hyperactive a stimulant, but these medications work *because* they increase dopamine and norepinephrine levels, giving the brain the stimulus it craves, and your brain no longer needs to seek out and create *additional* stimuli to feel good.

The most common side effects are decreased appetite and unhealthy sleep habits (like forgetting to eat, or not feeling tired and staying up past 2:00 a.m. most nights). This can become a bigger problem because physical hunger and mental fatigue can exacerbate *all* your ADHD symptoms. Just think about all the people you know who don't have ADHD: when they're sleep-deprived and haven't eaten in a while, they'll often feel distracted, impatient, forgetful, impulsive, and overwhelmed (typical ADHD symptoms)—so you can imagine the impact for a person who actually *does* have ADHD, who got only four hours of sleep last night and hasn't eaten all day! If you are taking stimulant-based medications, you will need to find strategies to make sure you're eating well and getting the amount of sleep that is optimal for you *regardless of how tired or hungry you feel or don't feel.*

Non-Stimulants

Non-stimulants are commonly prescribed for those who are unable to take or have experienced negative side effects with stimulants, and they can also be prescribed in conjunction with a stimulant medication.

One of the benefits of ADHD medication is that it can really help people stay focused; *however*, it doesn't help you stay focused on the "right" things.

People react differently to medications, so getting the right type of medication and the right dose for your specific brain and body can often be an exercise in trial and error, and you'll need to be the one to update your physician on how well it's working (or not) during your follow-up appointments. If your medication makes you feel like a jittery mess and unable to sleep, or alternately, if you don't feel *any* effect at all after a week or two, you need to let them know. Or if you're having terrible side effects, you may need a different medication altogether. Which is one (obvious) reason why you should get your prescription from your doctor and not your college roommate, best friend, or work colleague.

Less, But Better

When I was initially diagnosed with ADHD, my doctor gave me a prescription for what's considered a "very low" adult dose of a common ADHD medication. I took it as prescribed for six days and honestly thought I was going to lose my mind! I couldn't eat, sleep, or work. I was focused, though! I was incredibly focused on the most irrelevant things for hours on end and got absolutely nothing done. Even talking to people was difficult. My friends told me I seemed a bit "out of it," and when I spoke, almost everything I said came out at the wrong time, sounding louder and more abrasive. I stopped taking that medication and never tried anything else for years. (I'm extremely sensitive to medications and normally don't take anything, even for headaches.) So, when I was ready to try ADHD medication again, it turns out that I'm best with the smallest "pediatric" dose. My doctor didn't even know such a small dose was available, but I asked about it, and it is, and it works perfectly for me.

So keep working with your doctor to find the medication and dosage that's right for *you*.

What If I Don't Take Medication?

There are many reasons you might not want or be able to take medication for your ADHD. You may hate the side effects or worry about long-term impact or dependency. You might be pregnant and taking a break from your medication. There may be logistical issues like a shortage, or these medications may not be available where you live. Your personal preference may be to follow a holistic route, or you may not be interested in taking this type of medication ever—period.

Whatever the reason, even without medication, your ADHD symptoms can be managed once you learn the right skills. About one-third of our ADHD coaching clients have never taken any ADHD medication at all and are able to accomplish what they want with the right help!

RESULTS THAT LAST A LIFETIME

Regardless of whether you take medication, it's essential to learn new behaviors, skills, and habits that are designed to work with how your brain works! But learning these skills to help us deal with our symptoms, and building lifelong habits that will make our lives run more easily and feel a hundred times better, takes time, commitment, and practice. Which can be extremely frustrating for most of us who were born super impatient because we all want huge results yesterday!

But here's the thing: no matter how old you are—thirty-seven, seventy, or seventeen—you've had ADHD *every single day* of your entire life! So, for the sake of your sanity, your happiness, and your future, when you're learning skills that will change your life for the better, give yourself time to really learn them—even one full year is a tiny fraction of the time you've been dealing with ADHD! Don't give up on yourself or think you're failing because your entire life hasn't turned around after just a few weeks.

If you're looking for professional help, make sure to find someone with a profound understanding of ADHD who will tell you exactly what you need to do and have the strength to call you out on your brilliant (and believable!) excuses. The nonmedical part of your ADHD management program should combine psychoeducation, kinesthetic learning techniques, mood and life management coaching, proactive habit formation strategies, the right proven productivity tools (which are sometimes counterintuitive and the opposite of the tools that work for neurotypical people), and an expert level of ADHD knowledge and experience—all wrapped up in a directive and kick-butt approach with a ton of love.

Ultimately, regardless of whether you take medication for ADHD or not, you will always benefit from learning new approaches that will help you thrive in the non-ADHD world we live in. And, as a bonus for your time and effort, your new skills will never have a supply shortage, they'll never expire, and once you know them, they will last forever.

5

Women's Unique Challenges with ADHD

THE GENDER GAP

Even today, ADHD in women is under-recognized, and we are *still* almost twice as likely to go undiagnosed or misdiagnosed.[2] This being the case, many girls and women with ADHD suffer in silence and confusion, flying completely under the radar for their entire lives, their invisible symptoms making everything they do more difficult.

Both as children and adults, we often feel misunderstood, struggle to fit in socially, find it challenging to make and keep friends, and generally feel as though we're operating on a completely different wavelength than everyone else. These girls often grow into intelligent women living unbelievably stressed-out, lonely, and frustrating lives—achieving well below their potential despite their exhaustive efforts. They never accomplish what they are capable of and deserve, feel discontented and overwhelmed nearly every moment of every day, and worse, have chronically low self-esteem.

INVISIBLE EMOTIONAL CHALLENGES

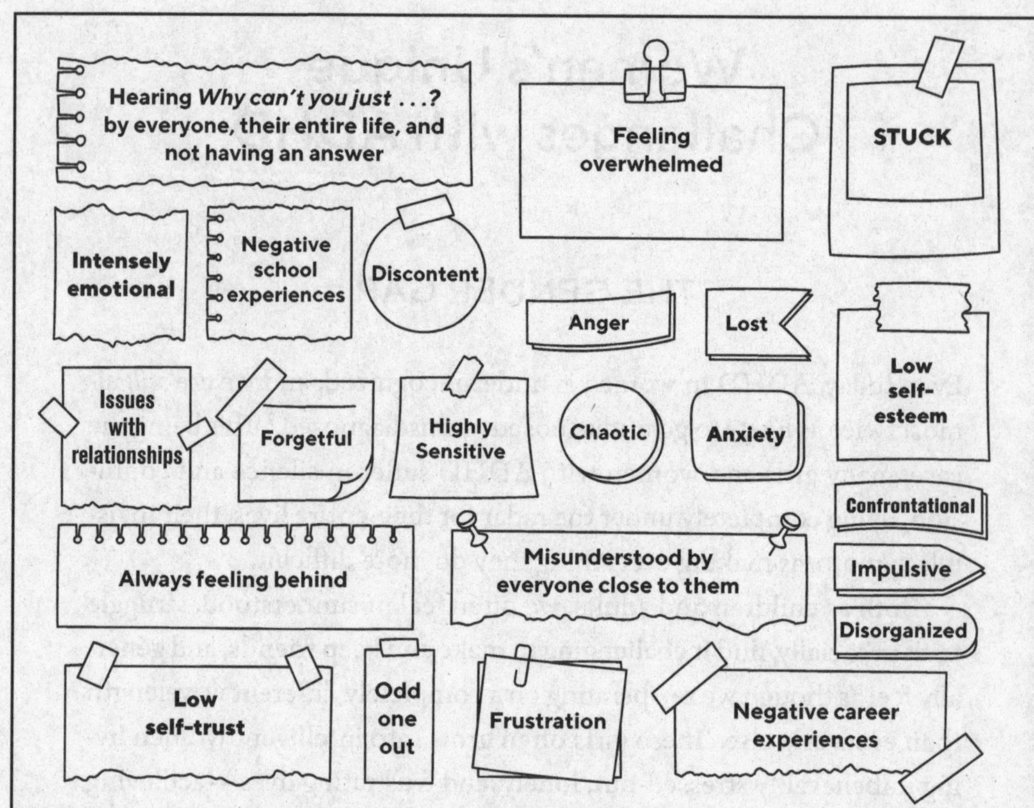

Relationships Can Be Hard—Really Hard

Growing up, many of us who struggled to read social cues and make friends in school also struggled with primary relationships at home with our siblings and parents, who also never seemed to understand why their daughter or sister with ADHD (still) behaves the way she does. On one hand, because of our history of not feeling accepted or like we belong *anywhere,* even at home with our family, many of us are hesitant to trust and more wary of entering into close, intimate relationships. But when we're in, we tend to be all in, particularly if we feel that we've found someone who *finally* understands us—that is, until we begin to second-guess ourselves, which will likely happen eventually.

On the other hand, because of our brains' need for stimulus, commitment to the same person over longer periods of time can also be challenging. When the brain is seeking out new and interesting input, it is often hard to be completely present with—and committed to—partners, friends, or family. There is always something to distract you from what's right in front of you. Which is why you may be averse to commitment. Sound confusing? Welcome to the world of ADHD!

Many of us also tend to experience more upheaval in our relationships and be more easily triggered, leading to outsize reactions to perceived criticisms. We find it difficult to remain in the calm, neutral zone for long because it's simply less interesting than the alternative. So, when things are "too quiet," we may subconsciously or unintentionally jack things up a notch by stirring up conflict!

Another severe challenge many women with ADHD experience is rejection sensitivity dysphoria (RSD)—which is an extreme and significantly heightened emotional reaction to feeling rejected, or the fear of *possibly* being rejected. A hypersensitivity to perceived criticism, even when there is none, can send a woman, who was otherwise having a relatively decent day, into a full-on panicked spiral of upset and excessive negative self-talk that can last for days or weeks. Sometimes it's so severe that they avoid all social situations to stay safe from interacting with others and potentially feeling rejected.[3]

Emma—Learning to Cope with Rejection

Emma is a savvy real estate lawyer with ADHD, in her fifties, who was unable to detach from a relationship that had ended years ago. Emma's self-worth was so tightly wrapped around her relationship with her ex-partner that she totally lost the person she once was. When the relationship failed, Emma felt she was a failure in life.

And when she learned that this man she had loved and lost was engaged to be married she was so crushed, she described it as "going through the trauma of death." She tried to keep her mind off him with endless activities, but nothing worked, and she couldn't stop thinking about how unworthy and unlovable she must be to have been so utterly rejected, adding to her frustration, annihilating her self-confidence, and holding her back from the possibility of meeting someone new.

After living like this for five years, Emma came to us for help. As part of her ADHD management, I immediately started working with her to break her pattern of distracting herself from her devastating emotions. By working so hard to avoid them, she had paradoxically ensured that they stayed front and center in her mind. Instead, I had Emma focus intently on what she had lost, and the many different meanings she attached to her negative thoughts. Once she was able to understand her subconscious need to hold on to these negative—yet stimulating—emotions, she was able to separate herself from the relationship, recognize that she matters a tremendous amount, is successful in many areas of her life, and, in fact, is not *a failure. The approaches she has learned over time have also helped her feel less hypersensitive to other real, and imagined, rejections so that now she is able to see hope for a new relationship.*

Living with Low Self-Esteem and Impostor Syndrome

Beyond our challenges with interpersonal relationships, we tend to overlook the struggles we face in our relationship with ourselves. This is especially prevalent for many high-achieving women navigating their careers. No matter how much time you've devoted to your education, the depth of your experience, your incredible skills, or the extent of your training, your success can still feel like a fluke! You may experience an underlying feeling that you will be "found out" by coworkers or supervisors, and at any moment, you'll be called into a meeting and be told that you're fired. Some women get into a habit of quitting job after job, even when things are going great, in the belief that it's easier to "get out before being found out." Since ADHD goes hand in hand with low self-esteem and insecurity, feelings of unworthiness, self-doubt, or distrust in your well-deserved success are almost never an accurate reflection of your true abilities or performance.

Mariah—Breaking Free of Impostor Syndrome

Like many busy women, Mariah was caught up in a cycle of overcommitting and overworking. Although she worked hard at her job, it never felt like it was enough. If only she could work harder and get more things done in a day, then maybe she would feel worthy. Deep down, she yearned to be understood and accepted by others, yet she felt like a fraud. She went through her day beating herself up over unread emails, messages piling up, and anything else she hadn't been able to complete in the last twenty minutes. Her negative self talk was relentless, as well as distracting. Unfortunately, the more unqualified she felt, the more her self-doubt interfered with her actions, paralyzing her further. She had lost all hope of moving forward with her goals.

To overcome her pervasive feeling of not being deserving or capable enough, we helped Mariah establish systems to regularly remind her brain that yes, she was responsible for some truly important accomplishments. Together, we carefully went through her specific achievements from the past three years and examined every detail of how she overcame the obstacles she faced. This helped to re-shape her self-perception by anchoring it in undeniable facts that were impossible for her brain to negate. As she kept these fact based messages front and center, and gradually internalized them, she slowly stopped feeling like such a fraud.

THE ESTROGEN EFFECT

Because estrogen plays a key role in regulating dopamine levels in the female brain, and women with ADHD have naturally lower dopamine levels and poor emotional regulation to begin with, fluctuating estrogen and other hormones significantly affects your already challenging ADHD symptoms and sets the stage for a colossal roller coaster of extreme moods throughout your life.

In fact, it's fair to say that the *constant* fluctuation of hormones that women experience every single month (for close to forty years!), in addition to huge hormonal shifts during pregnancy, perimenopause, and menopause—essentially throughout our entire lifespan—puts women with ADHD at a major disadvantage compared to men with ADHD, who experience far fewer hormonal changes.

During **PMS**, our ADHD symptoms often worsen because of decreasing estrogen levels, which can also explain why conditions like PMDD—a highly intensified form of PMS—affect women with ADHD about one and a half times more than non-ADHD women![4]

Pregnancy can also amplify our ADHD challenges, turning the emotional roller coaster of this time into an emotional rocket ship. "Pregnancy brain" becomes "ADHD-pregnancy brain"—especially if you've had to stop taking your ADHD medication. The rapid post-pregnancy decrease in estrogen can lead many women to report worsening ADHD symptoms at the exact same time that their entire lives are flipped upside down with their new (and beautiful) responsibilities. Sadly, women with ADHD are also up to five times more likely to suffer from postpartum depression and anxiety.[5]

By the time we reach **menopause**, estrogen levels decrease by up to 65 percent(!), with the accompanying effect on our dopamine levels, triggering intense mood swings, focus issues, and a worsening of

ADHD symptoms. Many women report this stage of life to be their most challenging, as the coping mechanisms that served them well throughout their entire lives effectively stop working. This exacerbation of symptoms often leads women who never suspected they had ADHD to seek a diagnosis for the first time in their fifties or sixties.

As a woman with ADHD, you are impacted by unique challenges—everything from getting a proper diagnosis, to coping with the impact of regular hormone fluctuations, to the intensity of living in a constant deluge of overwhelm, to the emotional impact that ADHD has on every single area of your life.

At least there's one thing we can all agree on: having ADHD is never boring! Especially when you consider one of the most fundamental ways it affects our lives—through our constant, often unconscious pursuit of stimulus, and the ingenious ways we create it *everywhere*, which we'll be looking at next.

PART II

Unconsciously Creating Stimulus

You'd be hard-pressed to find a warning on any description of ADHD that includes "may cause drowsiness." Nearly every common ADHD symptom amplifies excitement, interest, and intensity in our lives, and none of our symptoms ever cause relaxation, calm, tranquility, or any other term you'd associate with a spa getaway.

Our brains are wired to constantly seek out novelty, leaving us immersed in a whirlwind of nonstop stimulus creation, usually without our ever realizing it. This section will look at common stimulus-creating symptoms, most of which are rarely, or never, discussed, yet they impact everything in our lives from relationships to professional success to our personal happiness.

6

We ♥ Drama

I got off a plane in Amsterdam with $4,000 in my bank account (my entire life savings), a sixty-pound backpack on my back, and no idea where I was going to sleep that night. My friend and I planned to spend a few months traveling Europe by train and quickly figured out that we could save money and make it more exciting by hopping trains, hitchhiking, sleeping under the stars (or in empty buildings on construction sites if we were in a town), and basically living in a way that would completely terrify me if my own kids ever did the same thing.

Six months of traveling soon became a year, and we decided to head into Egypt. We could've done this easily by taking a bus, but "easy" was boring, and why be boring? My entire life had been spent avoiding boredom and I wasn't about to change that now. It was more interesting to go "off route," which for us meant walking across the border, sneaking aboard trains, and hiding in the tiny train bathrooms when it was time for tickets to be checked.

On the second train, we woke up in the middle of the night to find that at the previous stop, all the other civilian passengers had gotten off, and in their place were twenty big bearded men in camouflage gear with giant automatic rifles strapped to their backs, all shouting at us in Arabic to surrender our passports. We did. It turns out we had stayed on the train past the end of the line where civilians were allowed and were now in an off-limits military zone.

Eventually, the train reached its final destination—leaving us stranded in a remote desert outpost right on the border of

Libya. There were no other humans in sight except for the group of armed men who were still shouting and gesturing loudly, likely "discussing" what to do with us. We stood, terrified, watching as the train departed and one of the soldiers walked away carrying our passports.

My recklessness and impulsivity had landed me in the most dangerous situation I had ever faced as a woman. Images were flashing through my mind of my parents and grandparents back home, not hearing from me ever again, then finding out that I'd been killed and left to rot in the desert.

All in the name of my never-ending quest for stimulus.

After a while, a man in a white kaftan approached us and through gestures and pictures he drew in the sand, communicated that we had to go with him. He took us to his tiny one-room hut, where he gave us a place on the floor to sleep and for the next five days (it felt more like fifty), we stayed in hiding with his wife, who wasn't allowed to speak to us. On the sixth day, he returned with our passports and, a few hours after dark, walked us back to the train stop and waited until we were aboard, this time with tickets, heading to Alexandria.

LIGHTS, CAMERA, ACTION

Everyone loves a little drama. Our love of drama keeps us on the edge of our seats, needing to find out what happened to our favorite character on our favorite show or wanting to finish the book we're reading even though it's 1:30 a.m. and we need to wake up early. We enjoy the dramatic, beat-the-buzzer end to a sporting event, or a literal drama onstage. It's all entertaining, absorbing, exciting, and it keeps us highly engaged.

But for so many women with ADHD, drama seems to follow us *everywhere* we go, with relationship turmoil, job turmoil, life turmoil—or all three at once! Our lives can feel like a series of cliffhangers, where we wake up each day to find ourselves wondering what's going to happen next. It can be exciting, and there's nothing inherently wrong with it, unless it's creating negativity and stress, or holding us back—which it often does.

For so many women with ADHD, drama seems to follow us *everywhere* we go, with relationship turmoil, job turmoil, life turmoil—or all three at once!

If your life seems more dramatic than most, if there's more upheaval, more intrigue, or more stress than everyone else you know, rest assured you are not alone. Your brilliant ADHD brain has a legitimate need to increase the drama in your life, and when it doesn't come along on its own, we feel its absence, so we'll inadvertently create it. This can be seen as stirring things up or getting into trouble, or constantly moving from relationship to relationship, or from place to place. Even our friendships can be in flux. In general, much of our lives seems to be operating at a higher level of intensity than other people's.

We are not necessarily looking for drama, but it usually finds us. There has always been an inner restlessness inside of us and consequently, as adults, we attract what I call "high-frequency" experiences, which, although largely unconscious, are very effective ways to give our ADHD brain the stimulus it seeks.

Allergic to Boredom

Along with the old "Why can't you just . . . ," many of us may have been referred to as overly dramatic at some point. When we show up late to meet friends, before we have a chance to speak, we are greeted with a chorus of "What happened this time?" as if everyone seems to already know there is going to be a crazy story. Which there usually is.

You might not *feel* like you are manufacturing drama, but deep down, you probably know that the one commonality among all your many upsetting, totally random, or mind-blowingly "unbelievable!" experiences is . . . you.

We attract what I call "high-frequency" experiences, which, although largely unconscious, are very effective ways to give our ADHD brain the stimulus it seeks.

Not that you'd necessarily want a more predictable life. In fact, it's the opposite. You may look at other people and wonder, *How can they all be okay with the same thing day after day?* Too much predictability would be boring beyond belief, and for many of us, boredom feels like the kiss of death and must be avoided at all costs.

Breaking Up with Boredom

I was once engaged to a man who I can only describe as my parents' dream future son-in-law. He was a caring, successful, tall, attractive doctor. He took me on exciting, lavish trips I could never have afforded on my own and was the perfect picture of exactly what I thought I should want in a future husband. As our wedding drew closer and closer, though, I started to get cold feet. I genuinely cared for him, but some undefinable ingredient was missing—and I had no idea what it was except that it felt unnerving. When it came down to it, he was, well, boring. (As my best friend insightfully pointed out, "What do you expect? He's an anesthesiologist—he literally puts people to sleep for a living!") It's embarrassing to admit that the excitement about the lifestyle I was living with him had completely distracted me from his personality for over two years.

There was absolutely nothing wrong with him on paper, but when I thought about the reality of what it would be like to spend the rest of my life with him, it felt disturbingly predictable, in reality more like a nightmare, like being trapped in my own version of The

Stepford Wives. *The fact that he wanted us to live in suburban Connecticut and for me to stay home with our future kids and not have a career didn't help. When the day came for me to finalize our invitations, I panicked and called off the wedding—which caused a bit of drama itself.*

A Thousand Steps Ahead

Although you may not realize it, for many of us, the mere thought of stillness is so uncomfortable that it can actually fuel some of the drama in our lives. There's a sense of *needing* to be moving fast even if we're physically in one place, like sitting on our couch. It's as if our internal reality is always a thousand steps ahead and we're perpetually trying to catch up to it, which, of course, is physically impossible since we're here in the present.

Our internal reality is always a thousand steps ahead and we're perpetually trying to catch up to it.

This experience is extremely frustrating and agitating and can sometimes make you feel like you're about to snap. So you're pushed to do something, anything, to make it go away. You want to interrupt whoever's telling a story (especially if it's boring) and suddenly blurt out, "Just get to the point already!" because you're already thinking about the ending or the next, more interesting story. Or maybe you've felt compelled to stand up in the middle of a staff meeting (even if your boss is explaining the launch of an initiative that you'll be involved in) and switch to a topic that is more interesting to you, because in your mind, you're already beyond this initiative—or this entire *job* already—and are deeply into the next and better one. Or you'll tell your friend to just buy the darker jeans already because you won't survive waiting for her to try on another five pairs because your mind has already been at the party you're both going to tomorrow night, for hours, when the color of her jeans won't matter. And you know you're being rude and impatient, and you might upset a friend, or lose your job (when you don't really have a better one), but even those negative consequences feel easier to deal with in the moment than the unbearable feeling of never being able to catch up to ourselves.

READY, FIRE, AIM

As someone with ADHD, especially if you are plagued by an unconscious love of drama, in addition to regular day-to-day impulsivity, you've probably also kicked up the impulsivity a notch in some of the bigger, more important areas of your life. In the middle of doing one thing, you get inspired to change it up and do something else, go somewhere else, or find someone else. It's always interesting, but your spontaneity may have also gotten you into risky situations that went from exciting to terrifying. My experience traveling through the Middle East in my twenties was just one example of how my own restlessness and aversion to boredom inadvertently led to extreme drama in my life, nearly resulting in a tragic outcome. But if nothing else, at least it was never boring!

HIGH-DRAMA LIVING

You've probably gotten into precarious situations that, while not involving soldiers and confiscated passports, emotionally felt somewhat similar. You may have been riding high only to experience a crash landing. Perhaps you've dealt with a relationship that was filled with constant emotional drama and you couldn't seem to break free of it, or you take on huge projects with deadlines that you face with no preparation. Or maybe, like me, you're drawn to risk-taking and impulsively get yourself into messy situations that go from incredibly exciting to not okay to potentially dangerous, and you've done it more than once. Meanwhile, other people who look at the whirlwind that swirls around you may call you irresponsible, flighty, self-destructive, or say some version of "What the #%!? were you thinking?" But more importantly, you ask yourself the same question! *What* was *I thinking? Why do these things (always) seem to happen to me?*

How We ♥ Drama

The stereotype of the drama queen is the person who blows into the room, commands center stage, and wants all eyes on them all the time. This is *not* the case for most ADHD women.

In fact, you may be exceptionally shy and introverted, but because of a need to avoid feelings of stillness, your life frequently gets stirred up and becomes more chaotic without your meaning it to.

Creating drama is, paradoxically, a form of self-soothing, which gives a boost to your stimulus-craving brain. Anything less than captivating feels stagnant, which is intolerable. You are unconsciously trying to problem solve by creating more interest for your brain but do so through behaviors that may seem a bit excessive to other people.

Creating drama is, paradoxically, a form of self-soothing, which gives a boost to your stimulus-craving brain.

Making Mountains out of Molehills

Everything IS a big deal—for us. Even in small, everyday situations, you jump at multiple solutions as if your life depends on it, and in many cases, you can jump too fast and too high. This kind of overcorrection can occur in all areas of your life.

The reality for the ADHD woman is that so *many* things can seem major, and the first place she goes when faced with any issue is the most extreme response. She may be reacting to an issue or situation that will likely blow over but feels she MUST TAKE ACTION NOW or something much worse could happen. If you ask her on a Monday morning about her weekend, she probably won't say it was "fine" but, for example, will regale you with a story of how her kid got in trouble at school last week so she spent all weekend looking for a new school in the district, writing a bad review of the current school that she's thinking *very* seriously about posting online, emailing the principal, questioning and defending what happened, and looking into a new therapist for her child, which her insurance had *better* cover. These may be valid responses in certain circumstances but are not necessarily measured responses to the situation she is currently facing. Doing all this feels logical to her because it might help "solve" her child's school problem, but it's likely a major overreaction. Taking things to the extreme may help her feel as if she has some control of the situation but may not get a better result and could actually result in the exact opposite. Besides, next week, it will be something else.

Creating Chaos from Calm

This tendency to overreact, however, may not pervade all aspects of our lives. The ADHDer who is drawn to drama may be completely calm and in control in some areas and the exact opposite in others. At work, she might be an extraordinary leader, make measured decisions, and be responsible for extensive future planning, and then in her personal life, she may be someone who, for example, juggles multiple partners because being with one person *All. The. Time!* is incredibly dull and in no way remotely sustainable for her. This is so common. I can't count the number of clients who have shared their experience of *needing* to "wake up" their life by having an affair, only to deeply regret it later. Some leave a long chain of broken marriages in their wake.

Many women with ADHD are also quite confrontational. When things seem quiet, the need for some disruption can spur us to push other people's buttons, and many of us find ourselves bickering, picking fights, or being overly argumentative in everyday situations with almost everyone we encounter.

These actions and behaviors are obviously not exclusive to women with ADHD but can be more prevalent due to our pervasive feelings of internal restlessness, which can partially explain why the divorce rate for women with ADHD is higher than the norm.[6]

Getting into OPD—Other People's Drama!

When your own life is not very dramatic, you may create more intrigue by fine-tuning your radar to other people's drama, only to be sucked into it at the expense of your own needs and responsibilities.

OPD in real life is almost always incredibly interesting, validating, distracting, and entertaining. It's a perfect recipe for what the ADHD brain craves.

You may find that you often get embroiled in your friends' personal conflicts and ignore your own relationships, the deadline you have at work, and anything else that you might shove onto the boring back burner in order to immerse yourself in the drama and excitement of whoever's situation is the most interesting that day. I mean, let's face it, beyond the availability of dozens of reality shows, OPD in real life is almost always incredibly interesting, validating, distracting, and entertaining. It's a perfect recipe for what the ADHD brain craves.

There is a certain amount of excitement and sense of adventure that goes hand in hand with living a drama-rich life, but the challenge is that some of the drama you are drawn to can disrupt something positive. You also may have difficulty finding what fits or feels comfortable for you because as soon as you sense yourself slipping into a routine of any kind, you suddenly feel compelled to shake things up a bit.

The problem is that living with a background of perpetual drama means that it's almost impossible to have a low-stress week (or life), which can result in a continual sense of unease without knowing why.

Most of us don't want to live our lives in constant chaos and upheaval, forever redefining ourselves or taking dangerous risks that hurt us and our loved ones, or jumping from one thing to another and never getting what we want. And we don't have to. You can learn to dial down the drama and find ways to channel your need to keep things interesting in a much more positive, less chaotic way.

7

The Emotional Roller Coaster

Being controlled by your "mood of the moment" is one of the most common challenges for a woman with ADHD—as well as one of the most pervasive ways your brain unconsciously creates stimulus! Your overall mood can change multiple times a day, depending on what you ate for breakfast (or whether you ate at all), how much sleep you got, the mood of your boss or your friend, or spouse, or kids, or the weather, or traffic . . . pretty much anything.

While everyone gets swept up in their moods occasionally, most of what women with ADHD do or don't do is based on how they feel. When your mood is up, actions and results are up. When your mood is low . . . results will follow. Sometimes you're way up there, super high on life, with outstanding productivity, achievements, and happiness, but then something happens, your mood plummets, and you get totally derailed and so does everything else! And you can turn on a dime—something else happens that makes you feel good again and you're right back to feeling like everything is great! Our emotional experiences occupy a larger part of our lives compared to others and drive much of our day-to-day reality. This makes things challenging, not only for us but for everyone close to us who has learned the fine art of walking on eggshells whenever we're around them.

When your mood is up, actions and results are up. When your mood is low . . . results will follow.

While riding that emotional roller coaster is never boring for your brain, ultimately, it's exhausting, because you're constantly overrun by situations that others seem to handle without much difficulty. You may have been super excited about a new job, a new friendship, something you wanted to do for your kids, an amazing business idea, or something you *had* to buy for yourself, but then, in what seems like an instant, along comes an upsetting distraction, and the excitement completely vanishes! When your mood changes, *everything* changes along with it. It's as if the big emotions you had invested in whatever you were excited about never existed at all.

Rachael—The Ever-Changing Entrepreneur

Rachael owns a landscape design business, is in a promising new relationship, works out regularly, and enjoys sunset walks with her beloved nine-year-old golden retriever. She's also a supportive friend, has a wonderful sense of humor, and often works from her favorite coffee shop, where she enjoys interacting with the regulars. On the surface, Rachael seems to have a great life.

When she came to me for help, she confessed that over the past few years she had been feeling extremely disappointed in herself and her life. Her remarkable talent in landscaping combined with her intelligence and salesmanship gave her every reason to believe that she deserved to have accomplished much more in her business than she had. She was getting more impatient about doing the work she needed to do and waiting to get the results she had set her sights on when she started her business thirty years previously!

It soon became clear to me that Rachael lives with an "all or nothing; go big or go home" perspective that has her constantly careening from high to low. She can run with her mood and pursue a new goal, but if something derails her, all that forward momentum comes to a screeching halt. She loves the idea of going with the flow—it's always interesting and unpredictable, but it's hard to reach your destination if your flow keeps taking you off course while creating new ones—again and again.

Eventually, we helped Rachael make the connection between her ever-changing moods and the up-and-down outcomes in her business. Once she understood the source of her inconsistencies, we were able to build some nonnegotiable structure in her day, including learning the art of delaying gratification (more on this in chapter 12) to train herself not to run with her current "mood of the moment," as well as reinforcing stronger emotional connections to drive her productivity. After a few months, she was able to work with more purpose and direction rather than letting her moods constantly steer her off course, and her personal roller-coaster ride became much less extreme.

SENSITIVITY

Many ADHD women hear phrases like "Don't take everything so personally!" or "You're so sensitive!" on a regular basis. I've yet to speak to a single woman with ADHD who doesn't describe herself as sensitive, but it ranges anywhere from being "fairly" sensitive to having severe rejection sensitivity dysphoria and living her life mostly alone, avoiding human interaction as much as possible.

Everyone can be hurt by slights or criticism, but remember: most women with ADHD grow up feeling like an outsider and thinking there is something wrong with them. We are highly affected by our perception of how others see us and often hear criticism where none even exists.

When someone gives you feedback or makes a comment that you *experience* as negative or critical, it can hit you hard, and you don't have the objectivity to consider that their remarks aren't personal. Deep down though, you believe they are because your interpretation of what they're saying fits so perfectly with your worst perceptions of yourself.

If your boss says that something you worked on was "fine," you might take it to mean that you didn't do a good job. Or when receiving constructive feedback, you can't hear anything positive and may react in an extreme way, like running off to cry, sinking into a negative state for days, or quitting before you get fired even though your job was never in jeopardy.

Your interpretation of what they're saying fits so perfectly with your worst perceptions of yourself.

It's often the same at home. Imagine a woman who wakes up in the morning, goes to the kitchen, and as she is walking toward the coffee maker, her partner comments, "Oh, you slept in today." What she hears is him saying she's lazy and irresponsible, rather than making a simple observation. Because she has been conditioned to hear the negatives about herself and what she's (always) doing wrong, it rings true and hurts even more. She'll become offended and upset. So of course it looks like she's overreacting . . . again.

Ultimately, people in relationships with women who are driven by their emotions can find themselves constantly on their toes trying to avoid setting off an emotional storm. If partners, family, or friends have difficulty staying on high alert every day, they may simply give up on the relationship. Or they might form a very thick skin and not react to her, hoping the mood she's in will pass soon. While this may avert a conflict in the moment, it creates constant strain and slowly erodes the relationship.

For the sensitive ADHDer, it is difficult to see the big picture because the emotion that is happening *right now* is forming an impenetrable barrier between rational objectivity and what she is feeling. Even when she is completely self-aware and can objectively see that she's being swept up in a storm of emotion and knows she should stay calm, she has difficulty navigating her way toward the stop button. The prevailing emotion wins the day.

Emery—Emotionally Immobilized

Emery, a twenty-nine-year-old, highly sensitive college graduate, was so overtaken by her moods that she often had trouble not only getting out of bed but taking a shower, getting dressed, or deciding what to eat. When her mood dipped, she called her boyfriend or parents to complain about how horrible her life was, and nothing they could say could make her feel better, which of course made her feel even worse. It was easy for Emery to mask her emotions behind a smile and put up a "perfect" front in social situations so that no one else had any idea of what she was going through, but in private, she felt like a complete failure, especially as she was unemployed when she came to us for help.

Emery's struggles with emotional dysregulation and heightened sensitivity seriously disrupt her daily life and most important relationships. She is highly reactive, easily overwhelmed, and, to make things worse, she doesn't have any close friends. Additionally, because she often "doesn't feel like" doing what needs to get done, she has a long list of incomplete tasks, mostly related to her job search, which reinforces her belief that she'll never be successful.

In truth, Emery is both smart and capable, and deep down, she knows it. But because she found it difficult to function and accomplish much of anything while living at the mercy of her emotions, she needed to start learning some mood management skills to turn things around.

In the beginning, I started showing Emery some very simple strategies to temporarily get her out of her head (and overpowering emotions), feel stronger about who she is, become less reactive, and get her to move forward—quite literally! Beyond revamping her sleep schedule, one of her favorites was, as she put it, to "take my brain for a walk." Rather than staying on the couch overwhelmed by an ocean of emotion, we had her separate herself from the environment where she felt stuck and go outside for a fast walk accompanied by an upbeat playlist that we created together. As simple as this may seem, this physical activity was enough to spark a tiny yet necessary shift in Emery's mood. Over time, we worked on learning and implementing more permanent habits to manage her mood that boosted her confidence and now allow her to take on her daily tasks (yes, at her new job!), trusting herself that she can get them done.

Being at the mercy of your moods can be engaging for your brain, as well as a habitual way of being, yet it can make you feel like you are on a runaway train literally holding on for dear life. But there are ways to step off the ride. Regulating your emotions takes concrete strategies and practice. That may seem daunting, but is easier than you might think (or feel). By becoming less reactive, you open the door to deeper connections by allowing others to interact with you in a more genuine, less guarded way. Ultimately, your relationships with life, people, and especially yourself will feel more positive and fulfilling. And your brain will thank you for it.

8

Forever on the Fence

Are you unable to make decisions? Any decision? At any time? This is another way you may unconsciously create stimulus! From something extremely important like a career move, to trivial things like what to make for dinner tonight (because you had leftovers last night and ordered pizza the night before and you are kind of in the mood for Chinese food, or maybe sushi?), to what to wear to that business-casual event that all your colleagues are attending and you mistakenly wore ripped (although designer) jeans to the last one, you are always churning in the same decision-making agony! And then, no matter which choice you finally make, after basking in the calm and relief of having made the decision for at least twenty seconds . . . you change your mind . . . again!

It could be that you're not great at making decisions, or maybe you simply have an expansive mindset and are open to all possibilities. It's likely a little bit of both. You may find yourself living with one foot in and one foot solidly out the door in almost every area of your life, standing on one side of a lush field of very green grass thinking that the other side is even more green and more lush. You wonder, "Why can't someone just tell me, once and for all, which grass is the absolute best and greenest?" And being indecisive isn't only triggered when you are faced with huge, life-altering decisions; it is where you stand (or sit) on almost Every. Single. Decision.

WHY, OH WHY, DO YOU DO THIS?

There are a several reasons why it's common for women with ADHD to find themselves stuck in "indecision mode":

- Not trusting yourself because of having made too many "mistakes" in the past.
- Being completely overwhelmed by the ramifications of the decision and what it may lead to.
- Being unsure of the level of responsibility involved in the choice at hand.
- Being noncommittal and wanting to leave all options open, just in case.
- Being constantly engaged with the stimulus of the background hum of limitless potential possibilities! In other words, whenever you're in the middle of making a choice, life is a bit more interesting because you are immersed in the anticipation of the unknown. As soon as a choice is made, that hum goes silent, and after a while, that silence can feel intolerable.

Being indecisive can extend to anything—not only critical choices. We can know, logically, that choosing what kind of ice cream to order really isn't that important, and we can be told, "Don't sweat the small stuff," but no decision seems small, *ever*. What if it's wrong? What would happen then? It's like when faced with any choice, every possible outcome that could result from the choice you make flashes before you in a nanosecond.

Whenever you're in the middle of making a choice, life is a bit more interesting because you are immersed in the anticipation of the unknown.

Melissa—Delayed by Indecision

My client Melissa was pursuing a master's degree in creative writing when she came to me. Her program required that she submit an essay or short story every week. Despite having hundreds of ideas, she was always late because she couldn't decide which to write about. She'd pick one, then quickly change her mind. Melissa wanted her professors and classmates to respect her work, so she aimed for excellence. However, her assignments were never on time, and her grades suffered as a result. She knew she could do better if she chose her idea sooner, yet she consistently spent the entire week on each assignment bouncing back and forth, trapped in indecision.

For those with ADHD, the decision-making process is compounded ten times over when all the pros and cons for each possible choice are buzzing around inside your mind—all vying for your attention, with the same weight and emotional charge. They *all* seem valid, and they *all* have the exact same level of importance.

CHOOSE ONE (OKAY, MAYBE TWO, BUT THAT'S IT)!

Admittedly, it's more interesting and, at times, entertaining to remain in indecision mode with the familiar background noise of the great not-knowing. Once a decision is finally made, all that stimulus, all that speculation, and all that what-if agony is gone!

But then what?

The relief of having made a decision can be fleeting. So, in your brain's search for some good ol' cognitive engagement, you can then be pulled into the stimulus of second-guessing or dwelling on *all* the ways your decision can go wrong. Now you're trying to make decisions about your decision, and you haven't even committed to one yet. But your brain is fully engaged, and it can feel remarkably comforting to be sitting on that fence again.

TRUST YOUR OWN JUDGMENT?

You can get used to other people not taking you at your word, but it's much worse when you subconsciously agree with them and don't take *yourself* at your own word.

Your past choices may have been guided by pure emotion and momentary excitement, which can feel incredible and lead to some of your greatest life experiences. However, those emotionally driven, in-the-moment impulsive decisions may have also resulted in outcomes that exhausted and stressed you out, results you know for sure you don't want.

When you have spent a lifetime mired in trying to make choices—committing to one and then changing your mind at the last minute, or you've made a million perceived mistakes, or not followed through on something because you hit a wall—you may end up not trusting yourself to make *any* decisions. And it doesn't help that there is a chorus of people in your memory letting you know that you have been inconsistent, haven't followed through, and that you're unreliable. Frankly, you can get used to other people not taking you at your word, but it's much worse when you subconsciously agree with them and don't take *yourself* at your own word.

In the face of all this, if you've had a history of making not-such-great decisions, rarely follow through on the decisions that you *have* managed to make, and believe that no matter what you decide, it will end up in catastrophe anyway, then why ever go through the agony of making a decision in the first place? Being faced with any choice can leave you feeling confused, full of self-doubt, and just plain exhausted, especially when it comes to deciding something important. In fact, many ADHDers unknowingly use perpetual indecision as a refuge from taking responsibility for making important life choices, or potentially making a(nother) huge mistake.

NOT KNOWING WHAT YOU REALLY WANT

Many of us feel that we spend our days living in reaction mode. It's like we're living on a tennis court with a ball machine spitting balls at us at super-high speed and we're spending our lives running around as fast as we can desperately trying to hit all the balls back over the net. When this is your reality, it seems impossible to take a second to think about, let alone know, what you *really* want in your life. And if you don't know what you ultimately want, then how can you ever make a decision, not just about important things but on the smaller steps toward the bigger things?

Maybe you've had a hard time making up your mind about whether you should accept a job offer or you're trying to decide if you should pursue a different position in the field you really want to be in although it doesn't pay as well. Or you can't pick a paint color for the bedroom, or what to get your friend for their wedding. Or maybe you're faced with choosing between buying the small house or renting the larger one with a great backyard. Maybe your relationship is in limbo—is it time to finally get married or to stay engaged for another two years? And if you do get married, should you move to a different, more family-friendly neighborhood?

Making any decision becomes daunting when you have a history of not trusting your own judgment, or your ability to handle the consequences, or when you're unsure of what you ultimately want—because, let's face it, *that's* hard to decide! Not to mention that it's always more interesting for us (albeit stressful) when we're in the middle of making choices.

If indecision is something that repeatedly gets in the way of reaching your goals or feeling content, there are strategies coming up in part 3 that can help you to get off the proverbial fence. You can learn to make choices, big and small, that will guide you toward achieving whatever it is you decide you want.

9

Expecting the Worst

A lot of us with ADHD have a hard time remembering the last time something came easily to us and over time we have become conditioned to expect that things won't work out. We feel like it's always been a battle to achieve what our friends seem to do effortlessly. It's never been simple, never automatic, and never *not* a challenge. Is it any surprise that we believe it's our destiny to struggle?

Unfortunately, this tendency to expect obstacles in everything we do may have earned us the label of being cynical or negative. Most of us are not, though—in fact, we can be super upbeat and exude lots of positive energy—but our experiences have led us to be "realistic" about what *might* (likely) happen or how things *may* (probably) go badly for us. It's a habit that has been developed over a lifetime, leads to overall anxiety and habitual catastrophizing, and seamlessly feeds into the ADHD brain's tendency to seek out stimulus, both positive *and* negative!

GETTING STUCK IN NEGATIVE THINKING

There is a saying in journalism, "If it bleeds, it leads!" meaning that the more sensational the story, the more people will be drawn to read it. People are drawn toward excitement, even (or especially) if it makes us feel upset or worried. Frankly, the worst-case scenario is much more interesting than everything running smoothly—the more twists and turns, the better. Would you be more likely to grab a newspaper if the headline says, ANNUAL REPORT HIGHLIGHTS LITTLE CHANGE IN

HOUSING MARKET, or the one that screams, HEARTBREAKING TRAGEDY: COMMUNITY REELS FROM UNTHINKABLE LOSS!

Frankly, the worst-case scenario is much more interesting than everything running smoothly—the more twists and turns, the better.

The woman with ADHD isn't purposely trying to cast a storm cloud over everything in her life. She's simply developed a self-protective tendency to anticipate setbacks. She believes that disaster can strike at any minute (because it seems to happen regularly), and she needs to brace for it. Which, although unsettling, is anything but boring.

Some of this type of thinking can be directed at herself—those negative thoughts that live and breathe in her head that tell her she isn't capable enough or lovable enough. That little voice—which can be deafeningly loud at times—can echo the statements that she's heard about herself from others throughout her life: "Why can't you just (*insert complaint here*)" or "You can't handle it; I'll do it for you" or "You're too unstable; You're too unpredictable" or "What the #%*! is wrong with you?"

Frankly, we all have a voice in our heads that can either be a cheerleader or a trash talker. And we can usually recognize when things get extreme. But when you have ADHD, the negative voice seems to be louder than the others, dominates everything, and feels totally true. Any setback can become your inner belief of how things have been and will be for you *forever*. When you feel this way, everything positive in your life gets forgotten and disappears beneath the weight of the negative belief that this is simply how it always is for you:

"I was let go from my last job, so I'll be fired from this one, too."
"My partner left me. I have no friends. I'm going to be alone forever."

The negative worst-case scenarios that are conjured up in your brain often don't reflect reality but still act as a deterrent for you to try, let alone commit to, anything "bigger" that might feel out of reach. This can lead to you feeling hopeless and thinking that you'll never be able to accomplish anything meaningful. This is one of the biggest reasons that women with ADHD can be misdiagnosed with anxiety and depression.

We've had clients come to us convinced *nothing* will ever work for them because they tried coaching or therapy somewhere at some point in their life, and it wasn't effective. Anticipating failure is like having an insurance policy against disappointment. If you don't commit, you won't fail—again. The expectation of looming disasters can keep you firmly stuck in place, never committing to anything, and making it extremely hard to move forward.

Anticipating failure is like having an insurance policy against disappointment.

Grace—Rooted in Pessimism

Grace works as a paralegal and lives alone. She is super stressed, feels isolated, and generally has a pessimistic view of her life. For years, her mantras were "What's the point?" and "Things will never change for me." She put all her energy into her job, to the exclusion of everything else, which is ultimately why she felt so empty.

For as long as she could remember, Grace had been caught in a perpetual cycle of overthinking and looking for what could go wrong—unconsciously keeping her ADHD brain highly engaged, in addition to confirming the negative beliefs she always had about herself. This engaging pattern was keeping her deeply stuck in pessimism and fear and inevitably led to her struggle with anxiety and depression.

When she came to me for help, she presented "concrete evidence" that nothing would ever get better for her. It took a while to help Grace see herself through a more objective lens. I encouraged her to ask, "If a camera were capturing my thoughts right now, what would it see?" Together, we created a cost-benefit analysis (see "Create a Cost-Benefit Analysis for Repetitive Negative Messages" in chapter 12) for her thoughts and beliefs. Through this process, she was able to see that there were legitimate benefits to constantly believing that things just won't work out for her. It meant that she never had to take any chances or take on new responsibilities. Basically, she could play small, stay safe, and by not having any expectation of succeeding, she could never be let down. However, by unconsciously holding on to these "benefits," she simultaneously kept herself trapped in extreme negativity.

When Grace learned how to understand what was behind her thoughts objectively and where she was (and wasn't) in control of specific outcomes, it allowed her to better see who she is and what else she could achieve in her life—far beyond her job. Letting go of pessimistic thoughts, as much as her brain enjoyed playing around with them, while embracing more hopeful (and realistic) possibilities turned out to be even more stimulating for her brain. This shift initiated the beginning of a much happier, more connected, and love-filled life.

Always? Never? But What If . . . ?

Living in extremes is much more entertaining for our brains than living in (yawn) balance. So, if you find yourself saying *always* or *never* more than occasionally, you're likely operating on exaggerated realities that reflect your *feelings* about a situation—not the *facts*.

"I'll never be truly happy."
"Everything is always more difficult for me."

Remember, you have a brain that's happy to grab on to the negative and run a big city marathon with it, and because things don't (*ever!*) seem to happen easily for you, it becomes automatic to assume they never will.

The same is true for those of us who get trapped in the never-ending whirlpool of what-ifs. In movies and TV shows, the what-ifs can lead to riveting viewing experiences. In the brain of a woman with ADHD, they typically lead to catastrophizing, resulting in her becoming completely frozen with anxiety and fear of the negative outcomes that will come true because they are *all she can see.*

"What if I apply for the job and don't get it? (Wait—what if I *do* get it?)"
"What if I never fall in love again?"
"What if it goes completely wrong and ruins my life forever?"

You have a brain that's happy to grab on to the negative and run a big city marathon with it.

This weight of all possible adverse outcomes can overpower anything that is good and happening in the here and now. Even if what's good has *actually* happened in your life dozens of times, you'll worry about what you'll do when it all goes wrong and, as a result, won't try to move forward.

SOME POSITIVES FOR THE NEGATIVE?

Although negativity has figured out countless ways to infiltrate your thoughts and pose dire predictions for your life aspirations, don't despair! There are perfectly logical reasons for why you do this:

1. When your brain is fired up with the infinite what-if scenarios about how anything can (and likely will) go wrong, it's never, ever boring. Which keeps your brain on its toes (if only it had toes).
2. When you complain or beat yourself up, you are also engaging in a self-fulfilling prophecy. If you think something will go wrong and it does—you were right! You also get to be "right" about being a failure or not reaching your potential or abilities—these thoughts have likely been with you for a long time and will feel comfortable and familiar, even as they keep you stuck and hold you back.
3. On the flip side, some of us will purposely use these negative messages to our advantage, because needing to prove our own dire predictions wrong can be a powerful motivator to take the steps we need to take to achieve something important.

Sierra—Defiant Achiever

Sierra is a bright college student whose greatest life aspiration was to outperform her two older siblings. She had been diagnosed with ADHD when she was eight years old, and no one in her family understood it—or her. When she was ten, her siblings tried to convince her that she was adopted, and for a while she believed them.

Throughout her childhood, she was continuously criticized at home because she was always forgetting things, behind on her schoolwork, constantly getting lower grades than her siblings, and basically not living up to her family's high expectations.

She felt she was smart, but she had begun to doubt her ability to accomplish day-to-day tasks and was terrified of what would happen to her after college (if she even graduated). Her fear of failure as well as her concern that her siblings were possibly right about her pushed her to use their perception of her as motivation, rather than let it define her. In her junior year, to help inspire herself during exams, she put an eleven-by-fourteen picture of them on her wall!

I helped Sierra learn and implement numerous ADHD-friendly time management and study techniques; however, the strategies that had the biggest impact and helped her graduate with an excellent GPA were the ones that challenged her deeper beliefs and expectations of herself—something she continues to work on every day.

The subconscious has a hard time telling the difference between what is real and what is imagined. When you focus on the negatives, you feed them with your attention and make them stronger in your mind. One of the keys to countering all this negative thinking is understanding that the thoughts in your head are being created by you and you alone, and the feelings they inspire, while being incredibly engaging for our brain, are not facts.

10

Overthinking Everything

I've worked with so many women with ADHD who are unbelievably smart—maybe even a bit too smart for their own good. What I mean by this is that some of us who already have a tendency to overthink things also have the incredible ability to dissect the most minuscule details and make things far more complicated and time-consuming than they need to be. It may sound tedious, but it's how some of us unconsciously create stimulus—turning the smallest thing into a giant mental puzzle!

Have you ever come up with an elaborate system for getting something accomplished but the system itself becomes so complicated (yet brilliant!) that you spend more time developing it than you do on the actual project or whatever you were supposed to be doing? Instead of implementing your perfect plan, you end up spinning your wheels, contemplating *all* conceivable possibilities and getting mired in minutiae.

When you're a woman with ADHD who also overthinks things, it usually spills into *everything*, so it may look more like analysis paralysis on steroids.

As someone with ADHD, your brain has difficulty compartmentalizing, so every idea and possibility takes up the same space in your mind as all the others, simultaneously begging for your attention. You might sit in the same position for hours, barely moving, completely engrossed in nonstop, riveting mental activity. To the outside world, it looks like you're not "doing" anything because no one can tell how incredibly consumed you are.

Some people might see this as our supreme ability to hyper-focus. Others could merely label it as our tendency to get stuck in "analysis paralysis." But it's so much more than that, because when you're a woman with ADHD who also overthinks things, it usually spills into *everything*, so it may look more like analysis paralysis on steroids.

ALL THE KNOWLEDGE AND NOWHERE TO GO . . .

Women who overthink or overcomplicate tend to be highly cerebral and get caught up in the intellectual exercise of the task rather than the outcome. You may research just about anything because the facts and information you acquire by doing so are incredibly *interesting*! It's engaging (and fun!) for your brain to absorb new information, solve problems, or delve deeper into a particular topic. I mean, let's face it, who doesn't love to learn as much as possible about things that really interest them? But it's just as easy to get drawn down a rabbit hole for two and a half hours researching how to care for a specific variety of houseplant that you don't even own as it is to think about an extremely important work project that needs to get done by 4:00 p.m. today.

For the ADHD brain, all information feels equally important—and necessary. The problem is that all this research and fact-finding eats up the time you needed to accomplish something.

PROCRASTINATION BY OVERCOMPLICATION

Women with ADHD who are challenged in this area also come up against the widely misunderstood ADHD symptom of procrastination.

You're certainly not putting off a project by simply flaking off, scrolling through your phone, or watching hilarious animal videos online (not usually anyway). But dissecting and overturning every little thing makes your task much more difficult to complete—or start in the first place!

Being immobilized by your own "over-complicationization" (not a real word, but it could be!) can also lead to additional worries and fears. You may worry that if you stop what you're doing, you will never remember to get back to what you're currently working on, so you stick with whatever you're fixated on and let the other things fall by the wayside. You may worry that if you don't do the thing you've been putting off well enough, you will end up looking like you really *don't* know what you're doing!

It's all a lot to deal with—especially when these concerns are centered around your self-identity. It seems easier to avoid all that judgment (from others, and more importantly yourself) and take as long as you need to make sure everything is planned exactly right and, well, brilliantly!

Even at the expense of never actually starting.

GETTING IT DONE . . . PERFECTLY

On the flip side of the self-esteem-busting statements a lot of us grew up with, some women have been told for most of their lives how much potential they have because of how smart they are! Sounds encouraging, right? But because being smart (and always being told so) becomes part of our core identity, mistakes are not an option. If we make a big mistake, what would that say about us? (*Can you imagine?*) By doing things impeccably, we reaffirm our identity as a highly intelligent woman worthy of respect. But the problem is that nothing ever seems perfect enough or gets completed to our satisfaction, and when our standards are so impossibly high, it takes an eternity to never even reach the finish line.

Theresa—Probing Perfectionist

Theresa is a business owner who does her own taxes every year. She's always been incredible with numbers, and if she could stay on track, she could probably get the job done in record time. But once she starts digging into the books, she starts second-guessing her bookkeeper's system (unless Theresa's doing things herself, she tends to second-guess everyone). She then tries to figure out whether the expenses are categorized in a way that makes sense to her or if she should reallocate certain asset categories . . . none of which have any meaningful impact on her profit or the amount of taxes she owes. With all the time she spends overcomplicating the issue, she could easily have made back in earnings whatever she's trying to save by acting as her own tax accountant. In this case, her need to do things herself, perfectly, and get it exactly right, became more important than getting it done properly as well as efficiently for the benefit of her business.

We taught Theresa how she could overcome her compulsive need for perfection and learn to trust other people enough to do certain tasks (inspecting but not redoing their work). Once she was able to let go of feeling responsible for every single microscopic detail, she freed up the time and mental energy to grow her business by over 30 percent in a year. She came to accept that having things done at 90 percent by others was preferable to her own meticulous but time-consuming perfectionism.

Highly cerebral women with ADHD almost never jump to a solution or conclusion quickly, and they exercise caution in all things. If we're working on something important, we can get completely absorbed in looking at all the infinite angles and possibilities and, of course, coming up with viable solutions and even new ventures for all those angles and possibilities. At times, it can appear to others as if we are creating new complications on *purpose* just to have another new problem to play with! But really, we're striving for excellence, which can also be seen as perfectionism—even if we aren't necessarily perfectionists in *all* areas of our lives.

At times, it can appear to others as if we are creating new complications on *purpose* just to have another new problem to play with!

Regrettably, this often means that although the quality of what we manage to produce is outstanding, we almost never accomplish as much as we want to, leaving us feeling constantly disappointed with ourselves and frustrated that we can't achieve more.

All this overcomplicating would be overwhelming for anyone, let alone a woman with ADHD whose brain already has a hard time compartmentalizing. And although your heart is in the right place, because you want to put your best foot forward, your ever-curious brain can lead you to the stimulus of chasing down and getting trapped in a tangle of information and potential problems (that you now get to figure out how to solve).

Ultimately, you can learn ways to break free of your insatiable appetite for new ideas and knowledge, free up your brain to get the right information you need, and accomplish what you have set out to do much more quickly, so that you can dive into whatever you want to tackle next!

11

Constant Confrontation

Feel free to disagree with what I am about to say. I know a lot of you will want to, and the strong-willed, beautifully opinionated women with ADHD who tend to engage in confrontations *definitely* will—it's a tried-and-true way for their brain to unconsciously create the stimulation it craves! Being embroiled in disagreements and arguments about nearly *anything* is such an ingrained part of how they communicate that they often don't recognize when it's happening, realize how regularly it happens, or, more importantly, see how destructive it is. They can suddenly feel a burning need to get a rise out of another person and respond with a negative statement or conflicting opinion. It doesn't matter what the topic is or the level of importance. Additionally, everyone is fair game: partners, family members, friends, bosses, colleagues, total strangers—and authors of books about ADHD.

Maybe you contradict people as a reflex because you need to stir things up, prove your point or, at the very least, to know that you're being heard? Maybe you have pent-up mental energy that has to be released onto whoever is nearby. Look, it's not like you're a contrary, disagreeable person, even if that's what some people call you, and maybe they have a point, but more relevant is that your need to be oppositional, contrary, or argumentative is deeply rooted in a lifetime of feeling less capable than others and at times feeling completely alone.

PROVING YOUR POINT

A woman with ADHD can often find herself engaged in debates about things that are totally inconsequential and have zero impact on her life. The impulse to argue isn't getting her anywhere or solving problems; in fact, it's creating unnecessary conflict and affects everyone around her.

She thinks she knows . . . and many times, she does! But her need to assert her knowledge and ability as often as she does can come off as antagonistic and abrasive. She is not disagreeing just for the sake of argument but because needing to be seen as right (and intelligent) is very important to her, even if she doesn't realize it.

> **A woman with ADHD can *often* find herself engaged in debates about things that are totally inconsequential and have zero impact on her life.**

Having a brain that works differently from others', growing up misunderstood by almost every single person in her life, and at times being completely disregarded can make her feel resentful (even as an accomplished adult) and thinking that no one *ever* understands, cares about, or respects what she says.

As a child, you may not have had the ability or courage to assert yourself, but as an intelligent adult, you can invest as much energy as you want into proving your point and being right. You come equipped with a lifetime of residual hurt and frustration and the ability to speak your mind—at any time! If someone says something you disagree with or you know is incorrect, you need to let them know. This not only validates your intelligence but allows you to assert that you have an acceptable contribution to make and, for once, be heard—and respected!

Plus, to be honest, it's always a little more engaging to win an argument than to just (yawn) be agreeable.

Amy—The Knowledgeable Know-It-All

You probably know someone like Amy. She is always embroiled in a conflict. She is not speaking to her sister or her best friend from high school, or she's angry at her neighbor, and she is in yet another fight with a colleague. She is a bit of a know-it-all and is so eager to prove her point that she acts as if she's always right and doesn't need to listen to anyone else. If she lets anyone express their opinion, she's happy to let them know how completely uninformed they are. She comes across as being "closed-minded" or "unyielding" much of the time with everyone in her life.

After thirteen years of marriage, her husband was barely speaking to her. They were partners in business as well as in marriage, and when they were starting out, it was the two of them against the world. But once the honeymoon was over and they began to settle into married life, both their business and personal lives became more challenging. Amy's confidence began to dwindle, and she started turning her persistent need to assert herself onto the person she was now spending the most time with—her husband. Amy's need to validate herself and feel respected was so deep and strong that she was incapable of saying to her husband, "Maybe you are right," even if she wanted to and even when he was.

One day, she realized that because of her oppositional behavior and constant need to prove herself, she was heading down a path that would lead to the only man who really "got" her, and whom she honestly loved with all her heart, divorcing her. She could see it all happening, didn't know how to stop it, and felt guilty that it was possibly all her fault.

Amy came to us in desperation to save her marriage. We helped her confront and acknowledge her profound need for respect and understand the effect it was having on her entire life. We then helped her learn strategies for communicating more effectively—without confrontation, and ultimately, we brought her husband in as an ally. She was extremely fortunate that he was willing to learn about what ADHD was like for her, trying to understand the reasons behind her argumentative and confrontational nature, and how he could support her. By letting her guard down and allowing her husband in on her journey, Amy was able to reframe her self-perception as well as learn, implement, and practice her new communication skills so they could transform their situation into a fight that they could win together.

Women with ADHD who gravitate toward conflict can spend hours of their day defending their positions, whether it's only in their minds or overtly (and loudly) with the person they're arguing with. It's as if proving a point equates to proving our entire self-worth, not only to others but to ourselves. It's survival! Which of course is engaging for our brain. Arguments also serve as a battleground where we can win, adding an extra layer of excitement to the mix.

Proving a point equates to proving our entire self-worth, not only to others but to ourselves.

You may have done this yourself. Maybe you get into arguments, bicker, or provoke others more than most. Not just at home but perhaps also with your neighbors, colleagues, friends, retail workers at the store who won't allow you to return the item you bought on sale, the person sitting in front of you on the airplane who just leaned their chair back . . . basically, anyone who causes you to feel disrespected. The trouble is, creating all this conflict, although it's engaging, alienates you from others, because even when you "win," you caused the other person to "lose" (a situation they will want to avoid in the future—potentially by avoiding you). The net result is that you can end up feeling unbelievably lonely.

Resisting the urge to engage in arguments, whether to stir things up, release pent-up restlessness, or to assert that, yes, you do know what you're talking about, isn't easy. But if you focus on having more confidence in yourself and in what you know, you can learn to communicate in a more balanced way that conveys who you are without alienating and upsetting others.

By exploring all of these prominent stimulus-creating characteristics of ADHD in women, I hope you've gained insight and understanding of some of the factors that may have held you back in the past. Now, it's time to claim your future! Part 3 is your guide to actionable steps that will help you manage the characteristics we've just discussed, as well as other pervasive and challenging ADHD symptoms! It's a road map for making the changes you've been seeking, while helping you overcome the obstacles that have stood in your way.

So, get ready to take action and get back in control of your life. Onward!

PART III

How to Manage Your ADHD and Achieve What You Want

This is where the rubber meets the road! Each of the following chapters tackles a common challenge for women with ADHD—many of which were mentioned in part 2—along with proven strategies that have helped tens of thousands of my clients manage and overcome them.

To get the most out of this section, remember: Reading *about* a strategy isn't the same as knowing it. We often believe we "know" something just because we've read or heard about it, but real knowing comes from DOING. It's the action you take in your own life that makes all the difference.

To help you take action, look for this symbol: ☑

This is your **"For YOU To Do"** icon, and you'll see it often! It highlights a strategy or tool to apply in your life. So, please don't just read it—do it.

Additionally, at the end of each chapter, you'll find the One

Focus exercise—a simple, habit-building action to practice daily for a week. This is designed to reinforce key concepts, one small and simple step at a time, so that you can gradually integrate them into your life for good.

Buckle up—this is where real change begins! Xo

12

Manage Your Moods (Even When You Don't *Feeel* Like It)

Of all the symptoms that challenge us, emotional dysregulation surpasses them all. It's so prevalent that you could say that ADHD, while definitely being an attention disorder, is also a mood regulation disorder. What we do, and how we do it, is almost always based on our mood and emotions, which, as you know, can change a hundred times a day: depending on how our clothes fit, whether or not a package arrived on time, how someone spoke to us earlier, the number of hours of sunlight today, and so on! So you can have the absolute best and most high-impact ADHD management tools on the planet, but they won't be helpful for you if you don't *feeeeel* like using them!

As you may know from experience, your moods can be up and down, and because what you do often depends on how you feel in the moment, your actions will be up and down, too—which means that your results will be up and down as well. Mastering mood management starts with the crucial step of knowing when and how your emotions get in the way of your progress.

MOOD MANAGEMENT FOR PRODUCTIVITY

You're probably aware that your productivity tends to fluctuate throughout the day. Maybe you're a morning person, or you're at your best after 2:00 p.m., or maybe you're a night owl and you can practically feel your brain turning on after 9:00 p.m.? We all have a personal circadian rhythm, and you can make yours work for you by consciously tapping into the power of your most alert, productive times.

MOOD SCHEDULING

Without exception, every ADHDer I've ever known has experienced huge benefits from implementing "Mood Scheduling" into their life.

Think about the times of day when you have more energy and generally feel upbeat. This is the best time for you to schedule your most difficult, demanding projects. Conversely, the time of day you have lower energy is when you'll want to schedule your easier tasks.

☑ It may seem self-evident to match your energy and mood with the degree of difficulty a project may require, but almost everyone does the exact opposite! Many people have the most energy at the beginning of the day but spend that premium time mindlessly checking emails, reading news, or doing other things that require almost no thought or energy. Then when it comes to doing the things that require serious brainpower and stamina, they'll get to it at a time of day when they're already feeling depleted.

To find the time where your mood and energy align, you'll want to pay attention to your natural energy rhythms so that you can accurately know when and under what circumstances you have more energy, and when and under what circumstances you don't.

For a few days (ideally during the first two weeks of your monthly cycle when you're less influenced by your hormones), monitor your energy and your mood over the course of the day. At the end of each day, write your observations in your notebook: When was your energy down, and when was your energy up? Where were you at the time? What was happening around you? What were you physically doing? Did you get a second wind early in the evening? Do you tend to feel sleepy around 2:00 p.m.? Note as well if there are days of the week that are generally more productive for you.

You can also include in your observations:

- What regular tasks are easy, require *less* thought, or are more automatic for you?
- What regular tasks are more challenging, require *more* thought, or tend to drain your energy?

Now, whenever possible, you can match the level of challenge of a project with the time of day that will serve you best by scheduling in your calendar your most demanding energy-drainer task during your peak energy times.

You can also use what you've learned about your natural energy patterns to decide when to stop working on a project and when to take a break (go outside, drink some water, listen to music, or go for a walk). Just make sure to set an alarm for when your break is over so you don't end up on a never-ending break for the rest of the day!

☑ Stay Future Focused Using the Power of Anticipation

For most of us, feeling anticipation of what's to come is much more energizing and stimulating than the feeling of already having what we want.

Imagine a five-year-old child the day before her birthday. After searching around the house for what seems like forever, the child finds a hiding spot containing a few gift-wrapped presents with her name on them! She shakes the boxes and tries to imagine what is inside. For the rest of the day, she can hardly control her excitement! In the meantime, she is doing all her chores with a secret grin and being extra good. Tomorrow is going to be amazing!

What words would you use to describe how the child is feeling?

Now fast-forward a few days into the future to when the child has already opened her presents.

What words would you use to describe how the child is feeling now that she's already seen and played with everything? It's likely that her emotions are mixed and possibly a little bit sad that it's all over.

Feeling anticipation of what's to come is much more energizing and stimulating than the feeling of already having what we want.

Anticipation and desire for something you want has a strong emotional impact that can keep you focused and moving forward. When you have something firmly in mind that you are excited about, it can make the journey toward that goal easier, including doing the difficult or boring things you have to take care of along the way.

An easy place to start harnessing the power of anticipation is to consider some of the things you want most—those beautifully wrapped presents in your mind. Everyone, regardless of where they're from or how old they are, has at least one thing that they believe will make their life better (whether it will or not). What's yours? Write it down in your notebook so it not only becomes more concrete but will serve as a reminder for when you need it.

What would you be excited to have or achieve?

- A closer relationship with your partner or spouse?
- Having the time to take an afternoon walk every day?
- A job that you *want* to work at every day?
- Being comfortable inviting people to your home?

- Being able to make it all the way through a killer workout without feeling like you're going to throw up?
- Being able to spend more time with your family?
- Having the money to afford those golf clubs that promise to improve your game?
- Being able to buy a car?
- A regular night out with your best friends?

When you focus on something you're genuinely looking forward to, your brain will be instantly reengaged, and you'll feel more energy to keep yourself in the headspace that helps you to stay with what you are presently doing, while moving toward what you want.

Staying future focused is the opposite philosophy of "being here now." Because a lot of the present can feel chaotic and stressful for people with ADHD, when we focus on the future and firmly position ourselves on the launchpad of *What's Next*, we can soar past the chaos and overwhelm of our present headspace and focus our energy on what we really want.

BUILDING YOUR EMOTIONAL REGULATION MUSCLES

Even if you feel like your feelings have feelings and what you do seems to be at the whim of every emotion, you can begin to strengthen your ability to manage your emotions with practice and consistency, just like building physical muscles.

☑ Strengthening Self-Control by Delaying Gratification

An easy and effective way to improve emotional regulation is to practice the art of delaying gratification in different areas of your life. This can be especially helpful if you struggle with switching gears, get consumed by your mood of the moment or, while working, you feel compelled to complete every minor detail of unimportant tasks before going to the next thing. These behaviors can keep you from getting to what really matters.

To start training yourself to let go and move on more easily, begin by purposely stopping yourself from finishing something *unimportant*—no matter how strong your compulsion is to complete it. For tasks that have low, or no, urgency, you can set a specific number or a time limit, and when you reach that "stoplight," stop. Over time this small but consistent practice will begin to teach your brain to be less at the whim of your emotional impulses.

Our client Bria was at the end of a renovation and wanted to attach all forty-eight brand-new handles to her kitchen cabinets at once, even though it would take all day and she had a work project that was running behind schedule. We limited her to only attaching four handles a day for twelve days, which felt like torture to her and was also "the best thing she's ever done" for herself. Within a week, she had become more disciplined and in control of what she would and wouldn't allow herself to do in other areas of her life, regardless of how she felt about it.

Create a Cost-Benefit Analysis for Repetitive Negative Messages

When we get upset, we tend to replay the same negative messages to ourselves throughout our entire life regardless of the situation.

If you look closely, you may realize that many of your emotional reactions to situations are habitual and have been on replay throughout your life. By evaluating the specific costs and benefits of these reactions, you can start to become more objective and better equipped to understand and manage your emotions.

For each of these seven steps, write your responses in your notebook:

1. Ask yourself: What are the **situations** that usually get me upset?
    - *For example: When my partner or kids are disrespectful and talk back. When I feel ignored. When I can't do something I really want to do. When I'm talking and it seems no one is listening. When something is unfair.*

    **Some people will notice a theme start to emerge . . .*

2. Ask yourself: When I'm in those situations and feel upset, what negative **messages** am I consistently telling myself?
    - *For example: I don't matter. No one respects me. I'm always making mistakes. I'm always on my own. There's something wrong with me. I'm never going to achieve anything. No one will ever love me.*

Repetitive Negative Messages: You'll likely notice that when we get upset, we tend to replay those same negative messages to ourselves throughout our entire life regardless of the situation.

3. ***COST*:** What's the cost of thinking about these messages?
    - *For example: I feel alone all the time. I feel like an underachiever. I'm staying small and holding back. I don't have what I want to have for my family. I'm never satisfied; I'm always unhappy. I never have enough. I'm stuck in a terrible marriage. I'm stressed out all the time. I feel bad about myself every day.*

4. ***BENEFIT*:** Here's where you dig a little deeper: What **benefit** do you get from thinking about these messages?—There's usually one or two benefits hiding in the background.
    - *For example: I don't have to be responsible. I get to be right about being a failure. I get to be left alone. I get to be dominated. Others do my work for me. I can stay in this space where it's familiar and comfortable.*

5. Now ask yourself: **What if?** Who would I be, how would I feel, or what could I be doing differently *if* my habitual negative messages and beliefs *never* existed?
   - *For example: With those negative messages gone, I'd feel calm, grounded, fulfilled, content, happier.*

6. Create an **opposing statement** for your repetitive negative messages.
   - *For example: People do respect / have respected me. I matter. There are things I do really well. I have people to reach out to. I'll eventually achieve something meaningful. Someone will / does love me.*

7. Write out a simple "**I am**" statement for yourself based on any/all statements in #6 above that resonate with you as being possible!
   - *For example: I am respected. I am loved. I'm someone who can make a difference. I am great at...*

These positive statements are more difficult and much less habitual for most of us, yet they're more true than the messages you've been telling yourself for most of your life. Do your best to take a minute to allow them to sink in.

PHYSICAL LIFESTYLE CHANGES TO IMPROVE YOUR OVERALL MOOD

For many of us, especially once we're living on our own, things like getting enough sleep, eating well (and watching sugar intake in particular), and exercise are often left in the dust. As adults, we need to get back to these simple, low-cost, low-tech, basic tools because they can have a *massive* impact on our overall mood.

☑ ***Sleep:*** As we mentioned earlier, feeling tired creates ADHD-like symptoms for *all* humans. Now add this to an ADHD brain and sleep deprivation will majorly exacerbate your already challenging ADHD symptoms. But telling a woman with ADHD to get more sleep is like telling her to "settle down" or "stop worrying!"—in other words, futile. Your brain is naturally drawn to stimulus and, with its amazing ability to stay laser focused when engaged, probably keeps you up much later than you'd like.

Sleep deprivation will majorly exacerbate your already challenging ADHD symptoms.

One of our biggest challenges with sleep is that most ADHD medications are stimulant-based and can easily keep you wide awake for a full fourteen hours or more. This means that if you're trying to get more sleep and you want to go to bed by a certain hour, you'll need to take your medication as early in the day as possible to make sure it's worn off by bedtime. It may seem straightforward, but people often forget, don't take their medication until noon or later, and then can't figure out why they can't fall asleep until 4:00 a.m. Then they'll wake up late the next day and take their medication late (again), creating an exhausting cycle. If this is an issue for you, you can set a daily medication alarm to remind you to take your meds as early in the morning as possible. Or you can try *piggybacking!*

Piggybacking is tying a new habit to an already established one, like putting your ADHD medication next to your toothbrush or coffee maker to remember to take it when you go to brush your teeth or make your morning coffee. Combining something you often forget (like taking your medication at a time of day that allows you to get enough sleep) with something you regularly do (like making coffee first thing in the morning) is a great way to incorporate it into your existing routine and establish a new habit.

If you usually go to bed after 1:00 a.m. and you want to reset that habit, instead of forcing yourself to turn in at 10:00 p.m. when you're not even tired, make the change incrementally. Try going to bed just twenty minutes earlier than you did the night before. Go to bed at this new time for a few days, then go twenty minutes earlier than that for a few days. Your body and your brain will barely notice the shift, and there won't be much physical resistance to deal with. In less than two weeks, you'll naturally gravitate toward bed at a more reasonable hour, and your brain will feel much happier!

☑ ***Eating*:** Being hungry is similar to feeling tired in that it exacerbates all your ADHD symptoms. When you have ADHD, especially if you take stimulant medication and you're fully absorbed in working on something, it's easy to forget to eat for most of the day. Then bam! Your blood sugar hits rock bottom, and your mood goes to a terrible place. Next thing you know, you're feeling lightheaded, it's 9:00 p.m., and you've raided your entire pantry eating a ton of food that's not remotely healthy, because you finally realized you haven't eaten all day and you're absolutely starving.

Establishing general mealtimes and remembering to eat healthy, high-protein snacks throughout the day like small yogurts, cheese, mixed nuts, or low-sugar protein bars, and staying hydrated can make a massive difference in managing your blood sugar levels and minimizing major mood fluctuations. Do your best to keep a stash of healthy snacks nearby and keep a few in your car or handbag as well.

☑ ***Sugar*:** It tastes good, but for the sake of your brain, and your mood, and everyone who's affected by your moods, get rid of as much of it as you can. Refined sugar wreaks total havoc on the ADHD brain. Many of us love and can even be addicted to sugary foods, but it throws you directly into a downward spiral.

The next time you end up eating a bunch of sugary junk food, try to observe what happens to your energy and mood, not immediately afterward but the next day.

When I've asked our clients to closely observe their moods after a sugar binge, over 80 percent notice that they feel irritable and much more lethargic the following day. Some have reported that they felt more anxious and almost depressed! If you're unsure if this is true for you, the next time you end up eating a bunch of sugary junk food, try to observe what happens to your energy and mood, not immediately afterward but the next day (or you can take my word for it).

By eliminating as much processed sugar from your diet as possible, you're setting yourself up for significantly fewer plummets on the emotional roller coaster. Try going as sugar-free as possible for at least three days to notice the difference it makes to your overall mood. For an already mood-dependent woman with ADHD, removing as much processed sugar as you can from your life should be nonnegotiable.

☑ ***Physical Exercise*:** You likely already know that when you exercise, you feel better, and your mood improves, but it can still be difficult to incorporate exercise into your day. It's not just that you're busy and lack time; when you're not in the mood, it feels impossible to get motivated enough to move your body, even a little bit—especially when it's so much easier to remain lying horizontal on the couch! Your best bet is to start incorporating small amounts of additional physical activity into your daily routine. Simple incremental increases in physical activity will have a massive impact on your overall mood and your life. Remember, the real objective here is regulating your brain; getting in better shape is just an added bonus!

One of our clients, Sharon, is a great example of how beneficial upping your physical movement can be. She's in her mid-sixties and was fed up with how dependent she had become on caffeine to improve her mood and energy. So I asked her to start taking the stairs at work (only two flights)—not to lose weight but to help balance out her moods over time. Within only one week, with the simple change of taking the stairs to her third-floor office each time she went on a break, she had more energy and was in a better mood at the end of the day than she had been previously.

If you're not very physically active, start adding small amounts of movement to your life at any time, every day. For example, instead of always going for the closest parking spot, purposely choose a spot that's farther away, giving you the opportunity to walk for an extra minute. Or stand up while taking phone calls. Or do a one-minute workout (yes, only sixty seconds) when you're on a break, or simply just get off your tush and stretch.

Bit by bit, these small, marginal changes accumulate and can have a truly significant impact on your mood and consequently on what you can accomplish in your day.

HORMONES, AGAIN?

We already have a hard time balancing our mood based on our brains' natural dopamine levels, but now, on top of everything else, we have to deal with the usual hormonal shifts that *all* women experience. So what's a woman with ADHD to do? While there's no quick fix for PMS or PMDD, there are steps you can take to minimize their impact. First, it's crucial to be aware of what you're dealing with. Then implementing specific strategies becomes essential to managing your mood despite your always-fluctuating hormones.

Jasmine—Caught Up in an Emotional Tidal Wave

Jasmine is super energetic, always on the go, and acknowledges that she's so addicted to stimulus that she feels uncomfortable with downtime. Throughout her life, Jasmine has been in situations that have exposed her to both extreme structure and pressure, and to abundant criticism—a demanding mother, years spent as a ballet dancer, and then medical residency. The negativity she experienced took its toll, and she often feels down about herself, is critical about her work performance, frequently questions if she is doing anything right, and often gets stuck in regret about past relationships that failed.

Unfortunately, all Jasmine's negative feelings about herself are put into overdrive because of her monthly cycle. About four days before her period, her mood completely bottoms out. She describes it as being caught in a tidal wave where she can't think or breathe and is overwhelmed with anxiety and negativity to the extent that she feels suffocated. And although this is a monthly occurrence, it takes her by surprise every time!

The very first thing we had Jasmine do to get a handle on her hormonal disruptions was to track her cycle on a period app and black out as much as she could on her actual calendar for the days where she already knows she will barely be able to function. By marking the dates when her mood plummets on her calendar, she knows when and what to expect and can simplify her routine ahead of time.

But the ultimate game changer for Jasmine is that she now has a clear visual on her calendar that shows her that there's an end date *to it as well! Knowing she won't be feeling this way forever has been transformational for her because it gives her clarity and strength when she is in the throes of emotional upheaval, feeling hopeless and like there is no way out.*

Tracking your cycle in your calendar will also give you a visual "end date" to look forward to.

By tracking her mood versus just tracking her period, we helped Jasmine set intentions for those days as well as implement a mandatory ten-minute morning yoga routine on her balcony, which became her go-to exercise to start the day feeling a bit more connected with herself. These habits (tracking when to expect her mood to plummet, setting intentions, and a simple positive activity to start the day) help her ride the wave of her hormone-driven mood shifts, not get as overwhelmed, and come out the other side.

The Three Rules of ADHD and PMS

☑ 1. Know in advance when your mood is going to hijack you (and your sanity) by *tracking your cycle* and *your mood* so that you are never caught by surprise again. Put a recurring "warning" note in your calendar in advance for the days that you'll likely be affected so that you are not caught off guard thinking, *What the heck is wrong with me?* when you are totally overwhelmed by extreme emotion. Tracking your cycle in your calendar will also give you a visual "end date" to look forward to, when it feels like it will never end.

☑ 2. During that time of the month, schedule *in advance* at least one simple activity per day that brings you some level of happiness and relief: yoga, baking, napping, dancing, strength training, snuggling with your pet, doodling, watching music videos, or talking to your best friend—whatever works for you. Even if you only do it for ten minutes, commit to one of these as a "must-do" daily task for this time of the month.

   * Go to your calendar now and input a few activities of choice on those days—don't wait to do it later when you definitely won't feel like it.

☑ 3. Set a rule to avoid making any major decisions during this time. Make a note to yourself in your calendar that says something simple like: "No Major Decisions Allowed. Seriously—None!"

By simply noting when your moods shift and what is going on when that happens, you can then implement at least one of these strategies and make conscious choices rather than being driven by your prevailing mood.

DAILY MOOD SHIFTERS: WHAT TO DO WHILE YOU'RE UPSET

Below are simple approaches that you can incorporate into your daily life to help manage the regular, more frequent negative emotions that can affect you every day, multiple times a day. These techniques have proven very effective for our clients when it comes to taking control of the negative moods that cause pain in their lives.

☑ Check Your Expectations

We can get upset for a hundred different reasons, yet it often comes down to something quite simple: our expectations were not met.

Play with this concept the next time you feel upset, no matter what the situation is, and ask yourself:

1. What did I want or expect that didn't happen or that I didn't get?
2. What if I never had that expectation?

Write the answers down in your notebook. Doing this will help you recognize patterns in the things that cause you to become upset (or frustrated, angry, or generally feel bad). And when you can identify a pattern, you have a much better chance of breaking it.

☑ Feel the Burn

When we exercise to build muscle, we work it *until we feel the burn*, pushing through the pain to make ourselves do a few more reps, and it would be very unusual for someone to build muscle without experiencing *any* feelings of discomfort—or pain. We can think about building our emotional "muscles" in a similar way.

Negative emotions have a way of spilling into our entire being and throwing us off whatever well-intentioned path we're on. Imagine if, instead of trying to push those emotions away (like disappointment, sadness, or rejection), you worked to push *through* them. When you allow yourself to acknowledge, focus on, and fully experience negative emotions, their grip on you becomes much weaker.

To be clear, I'm *not* talking about accepting negative situations (although you can, and some incredibly wise teachers say that we should!) but rather accepting the painful *emotions* that go along with what happened.

When you allow yourself to acknowledge, focus on, and fully experience negative emotions, their grip on you becomes much weaker.

When negative emotions bulldoze themselves into your soul, invite them in and feel them entirely—do your best to see them for what they are. Pause and try to notice where the negativity (or your automatic reaction) came from—your beliefs and expectations—then find the center of the feeling. Maybe it burns and it hurts, a lot, but just like when you're working out, you can feel the burn, acknowledge it, explore where it came from, accept it, push through it, and continue.

Fully embracing and processing an emotion usually takes less than one minute, and what often happens is similar to what happens when you stare at something intently until it begins to blur, or when you think about and repeat the same word or phrase out loud over and over again until it loses its meaning. When you remain intently focused on the emotion that's essentially hijacking your life right now, it loses its grip on you and will eventually begin to dissipate.

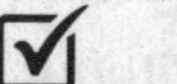

Mood Rescue Kit

You can't always anticipate when or how certain emotions will show up, but you know from experience that a certain time of day or a certain type of situation is guaranteed to pull you into a mood that can slow down or potentially stop your progress entirely. If you're prepared for these situations and have a couple of tools at your disposal for coping with them, you can help to keep your emotions at bay.

Think of this as your personal Mood Rescue Kit. To create it, start with a small bag or container that you'll keep somewhere accessible, like at your desk, in your room, or in your car. It will contain a few tangible items to use when you are emotionally stuck.

Items that have been most beneficial to our clients include music or a playlist—or a list of specific songs to listen to ASAP; a book written by your favorite motivational speaker; the names of two people who make you laugh and that you can reach out to; a feel-good keepsake; printed photos that elicit amazing memories; a poem or lyrics from a song; a printed copy of an email or text that made you feel absolutely incredible when you received it; or anything else that makes you smile.

For many of us, physical objects and experiences have a more immediate and powerful impact on our emotions than abstract thoughts. When you physically touch and see things that hold positivity, you give yourself the ability to alter your mood—even if only momentarily, it's enough to cause a shift. For many of my clients, purposely changing their mood becomes a habit, and for some, it also feels like a game that their mind really loves to play—and win.

Chances are, it will for you, too.

☑ Model Your Role Model

This exercise will take you out of your own head and into someone else's who, at least in this moment, is someone whose head you'd like to be in.

Choose someone you know well and that you look up to. A mentor, your best friend, a family member you've always admired, a public figure you've never met but respect deeply. What's their name? Why do you admire them? Think about them going about their day-to-day life for at least thirty seconds.

In your notebook, write down their name and make a list of their attributes: How do they behave? What would they do or how would they react in a particular stressful situation (perhaps one that you're in right now)? What do you think they'd be thinking and saying?

Pausing your own train of thought and putting yourself in the mindset of someone else entirely can give you a much-needed interruption from your own relentless inner dialogue and inspire you to think in a completely new and different direction.

MANAGING EXTREME NEGATIVITY

Some of us can get bulldozed by deep negative moods, and when they show up again and again, regardless of the situation, it's usually the exact same feeling, with the same message, forcing itself into our lives. You can try to ignore it and make attempts to focus on the positive, but it shows up and sticks around anyway, no matter how hard you try to push it away, leaving you feeling upset, despondent, and unmotivated.

I created these "not-so-simple" techniques years ago, and they've been incredibly effective for all our clients. You'll want to read about and practice them now, *before* you become swallowed up in an upsetting situation, so that you'll be prepared to manage your reactions and responses when you really need it.

NON-DOMINANT HANDWRITING

Writing by hand—especially with your non-dominant hand—rather than typing on a keyboard or dictating a voice memo is one of the fastest ways to force your brain to slow down and focus so that you can more fully absorb the information.

☑ Instead of being slammed by negative emotions and reacting on autopilot, the next time something happens that you find upsetting, take control with this three-step technique.

Step 1: Record whatever it was that upset you in your notebook, *writing it down by hand.* Accept any emotions that come up while you're doing this and let them in. Heck, feel free to welcome them in with open arms and offer them a snack!

Step 2: To slow down your beautiful mind even more, write down what upset you again, this time with your *non-dominant* hand. Don't worry about how your handwriting looks. No one will ever see this except you. Hopefully after you've written out the upsetting scenario with your dominant *and* non-dominant hand, you're in a less reactive, possibly slightly calmer place.

Step 3 (The Most Important Step): Now think of one or two potential solutions for what upset you, and in your notebook, write each solution out three times with your non-dominant hand. (You might notice while doing this that your non-dominant handwriting is getting a tiny bit easier! Look at you!)

Potential Solution 1: (Write it down in your notebook three times with your non-dominant hand)

Potential Solution 2: (Write it down in your notebook three times with your non-dominant hand)

Once you're in a more analytical mindset, instead of *only* stewing in negative emotions, your mind will be refocused on potential solutions.

STEP BACK TO FREEDOM

I designed the Step Back to Freedom technique to help women with ADHD manage the negative emotions that can become so all-encompassing they end up having a major influence on our lives. This is a visualization exercise you can turn to when you feel hijacked by a negative emotion and is also one of my personal favorites that I often use myself.

☑ To get started, get comfortable and think of whatever is upsetting you and the messages you're telling yourself about this situation. Whatever emotions surface, take a few seconds to allow yourself to feel them. Now, do your best to give the primary emotion—the one that's a little bit louder than the others—a name. Don't think about it for too long. Simply say the first word that comes up for you. Is it anger? Regret? Guilt? Shame? Resentment? Resignation? Sadness? Hopelessness?

Imagine that this emotion has a shape. Or, to make it more interesting for your brain, you could think of it as a cartoon character with a personality. (Thanks, Pixar, for making this part of the exercise much easier to understand!) Now picture the emotion's shape, or character, five feet away from you.

Now envision yourself backing away from it until it's one hundred feet away. As you continue to back farther away from it, you can still see the emotion as a shape that is getting smaller and smaller until it becomes a tiny image that you can barely see.

Notice how much immense space there is now between you and the emotion. Notice that this huge silent space is much bigger than the energy of the emotion you were experiencing.

Your emotion isn't you and it never was. It's a valid emotion, but it is not *you*. It is completely separate and is so far away from you now that it looks like a tiny dot. You are over here, with an expansive open space in front of you, behind you, and all around you. That emotion used to take up infinite space in your heart and mind, or at least maybe you *thought* it did. But by taking a closer look, naming it, and ultimately walking away and separating yourself from it, you gain perspective on what it is: one emotion inside a massive and endless universe of space and possibility.

Your emotion isn't you and it never was.

This is when you can ask yourself: What is possible now that the emotion became a faraway teeny-tiny dot?

Mentally envisioning separating yourself from your all-consuming emotions so that you can see them for what they are gives you much-needed perspective to choose your reaction or response, subsequently giving *you* the opportunity to not let them dominate you ever again.

ADHD-Friendly Quick Summary

- ADHD impairs our ability to *regulate* our emotions.
- Our mood of the moment tends to dictate our entire reality.
- Use Mood Scheduling to get things done:
  * High-energy times of day = difficult tasks and projects
  * Low-energy times of day = easiest tasks and projects
- Harness the emotional power of anticipation to stay motivated.
- Building your emotional regulation muscles begins with a small increase in self-control and becoming more objective and analytical toward your negative thoughts.
- Your habitual negative beliefs have costs as well as benefits. Know what these are.

(continued on next page)

(continued from previous page)

- Take care of your brain with body basics: more sleep, healthy nutrition, less sugar, and more physical activity.
- Hormonal factors that all women experience significantly exacerbate our challenge with mood regulation.
- Track your cycle as well as your mood so that you're never caught off guard again.
- Check your wants and expectations every time you feel upset.
- Accept and fully experience your negative emotions to diminish their power over you.
- Brainstorm and handwrite potential solutions with your non-dominant hand following an upsetting moment.
- Step Back to Freedom: Shrink your emotions down to size. Create a huge empty space between you and your emotions. That empty space is where new possibilities exist.

ONE FOCUS

Great Expectations Check-In

Start noticing how your expectations are connected to your negative moods. For one full week, every single time you begin to feel upset, ask yourself:

1. What was I expecting that I didn't get?
2. What if I never had that expectation?

Write down or make a voice memo of your answers. After one week, you'll likely start to notice patterns of the things and situations that cause you to feel upset, frustrated, or angry most often and the part that your expectations are playing. This can significantly help you manage your emotions when these situations happen in the future.

13

Simplify Decision-Making

While everyone struggles with indecision from time to time, many women with ADHD have challenges making decisions *all* the time—whether they're big or small. Our difficulty with decision-making comes in two forms. You might have trouble making decisions to the point where you can't make any decisions at all, and your days are spent in a constant back-and-forth dance with yourself. At the other extreme, you may make impulsive decisions, jumping at the first idea that pops into your head without taking time to evaluate the consequences. Or, you may do a little bit of both.

It helps to explore some of the reasons for both kinds of decision-making difficulties before getting to the solutions, and we'll talk about being stuck in indecision first.

FOR THE FENCE-SITTERS . . .

If you are perpetually indecisive, let's take a deeper look at a few things that keep you from getting off that proverbial fence. Hopefully, some of these will sound familiar, as we mentioned them in chapter 8 when talking about the unconscious ways we create stimulus.

Fear of Missing Out (FOMO)

Living with perpetual information overload can make it difficult to make one choice, especially when you can see 105 different pathways.

It's difficult, and sometimes torturous, to choose only one. It's like being a kid in a candy store—all the possibilities seem so good; how can you possibly choose? If you choose only one, you might get it wrong or miss out on all the other options that could be so much better! It's FOMO on steroids.

Playing It Safe

Many of us, especially as we get older, use indecision to avoid facing our fear of potentially making a big mistake or of being held accountable for a particular choice. Our hesitation often stems from not wanting to be perceived as being flaky, unintelligent, or incorrect, particularly if the decision affects our family, career, or other responsibilities—which all feel super important. It can also be debilitating to think about others who might be impacted by *your* decision. The more responsibilities you have, the higher the stakes can feel. So, while you do everything humanly possible to avoid making mistakes, ultimately the only way to avoid them completely is not make a decision in the first place.

All the Good and All the Bad, All at Once

It's hard to make important decisions when all the pros and cons are swirling around inside your mind at the exact same time, with the same weight and emotional charge. Every choice and every potential positive and negative outcome washes over you in an instant! How can you possibly pick one option under those overwhelming circumstances? With all the different possible outcomes spinning you around and around, you can tie yourself in knots trying to come to a decision, even when you logically know that whatever you are trying to decide is not *that* important.

A Matter of Trust

If you don't fully trust yourself, how can you trust your decisions? Perhaps you made a choice that didn't turn out well for you or others, or you missed a big opportunity because you couldn't make up your mind. You may replay those situations over and over, leaving you without much faith in your own decision-making abilities.

If you don't fully trust yourself, how can you trust your decisions?

Although you have made decisions in the past that turned out well, you tend to forget those, and only remember the bad outcomes. This lack of self-trust makes it harder to commit to any decision. And, when it comes to making important decisions and the stakes are high, you can be left feeling unsure, dizzy, and resigned to not moving forward.

Not Knowing What You Really Want

What if you don't know what truly makes you happy? Perhaps you have a hard time making up your mind about what career to pursue, where you want to live, or who you want to spend time with? Maybe your past choices have been driven by pure emotion and momentary excitement, and that led to some of your greatest moments, but it just as easily could have resulted in deep regret later. If you don't know what you want or what is really important to you, how can you possibly make the right decision—or *any* decision?

THE FLIP SIDE: IMPULSIVE DECISION-MAKERS

There is another type of decision-making challenge that's just as common and stress-inducing for us yet doesn't seem to get nearly as much airtime. I'm sure you are familiar with the phrase *ready, aim, fire*. Impulsive decision-makers completely bypass the *aim* part. Some of the reasons for those straight-to-action-without-much-thought, consequences-be-damned snap decisions include:

The Overwhelm of Too Many Options

If your brain is very busy with a number of options and you don't have enough time (or so your brain tells you) to evaluate them all, making rash decisions feels like a necessary escape, providing an enormous sense of relief. Plus, making those impulsive decisions momentarily feeds your stimulus-seeking brain, which also feels quite satisfying.

Needing to Know NOW

Many of us struggle with the in-between-ness and uncertainty of not knowing. It's as if not clearly seeing a destination ahead creates additional overwhelm that is so uncomfortable and so all-consuming, you will make a choice, any choice, right now, just to avoid that pain.

Escaping Intense Restlessness and Boredom

When boredom or restlessness sets in, it can feel agonizing, and let's be honest, for some of us, taking the time to think things through to make a well-thought-out decision is simply NOT doable when we're already thousands of steps ahead of the decision and feeling excruciatingly impatient to get to the next thing. We'll do *anything* to escape this feeling, resorting to making rash decisions and taking actions based on what provides relief in that exact moment. Many "What on earth was I thinking?" impulsive decisions stem from feeling like this.

Being in High-Pressure Situations

Impulsive decision-making is also common for people who have high-pressure leadership roles, are juggling too many responsibilities, or are under a lot of pressure from others to perform. It can feel more important to cross an item off their to-do list without much thought than to take the time to weigh it out. Sometimes this type of impulsive decision-making can be preceded by weeks (or months) of overthinking. Then, when the external pressure suddenly hits, we'll make a fast decision just to get it over with.

Impulsive decision-making is the polar opposite of being indecisive, but it has the same ultimate effect. It feels engaging in the moment but often lands you in situations that lead to additional work and stress, especially if it creates conflict with others who were affected by your decision.

HOW TO MAKE DECISIONS *FASTER* (FOR TEAM INDECISIVE) OR *SLOWER* (FOR TEAM IMPULSIVE)

Being in indecision mode can be interesting and exciting. Before a choice is made, all the potential possibilities create a rhythmic background noise, and once the decision is finally made, all that stimulus suddenly goes away, and it's quiet. The relief of knowing what to do feels absolutely incredible—for about fifteen seconds! But then the quiet in your mind begins to feel disconcerting and can revolt at a deafening volume through second-guessing your decision or by creating new decisions about the decision.

It also feels more interesting, engaging, and at times entertaining when you make impulsive decisions. These can keep you moving forward at a faster pace without having to think too much and can relieve any overwhelm and pressure quickly—just sometimes (or often) to your detriment.

Whichever scenario describes your decision-making, there are ways to balance out the process, so you are making solid choices from a place of knowledge and strength. The following strategies are tried-and-true favorites that have helped my clients make decisions, big and small, with much less angst and a lot more certainty.

Pick a Limit, Any Limit

Placing some parameters on your decision-making allows you to narrow your focus, cut out extraneous distractions, and zero in on what you want to do. These limits will act as a boundary for your brain so the choices feel less infinite.

☑ Limits for Team Indecisive: Narrow Your Options

***Time limit*:** I have five hours to make this decision; I have three days to choose which program I'm signing up for.

***Budget limit*:** I can spend up to fifty dollars on this.

***Limit the variables*:** I'm only picking something in a blue or purple tone; I'm only considering hotels that include breakfast.

***Numerical limit*:** I'm going to check the reviews for a maximum of five products before choosing one; I'll visit six universities before deciding where to apply.

By identifying a limit, you're putting yourself in charge and avoiding the possibility of becoming dizzy over a nonstop array of limitless possibilities for your brain to stress over.

☑ Limits for Team Impulsive: Decide Not to Decide

On the other hand, if you are prone to rash decisions, you need a different type of rule that will encourage you to take a time-out or delay your decision before jumping at an option. Think of your rule like a traffic roundabout that you're building in your brilliant brain to slow down the intense internal speed and pressure you feel to make a decision *now*.

***Hit Pause*:** No immediate decisions allowed, must pause for a minimum of ten minutes.

***Take a Breath (or Three)*:** Don't respond verbally to another person with a decision until you take three deep breaths or count to seven.

***Reset Your Brain*:** No decisions until at least the next day after you sleep on it.

***Check First*:** Hold off on making any decisions until you've completed a brief "decision checklist," which can include writing down factors like costs, risks, benefits, alternatives, and so on.

Use *any* pause method that helps you slow down, take a moment, and reduce the internal pressure you feel to make an instant decision.

Move from Emotional to Analytical

Do you feel you're terrible at certain types of decisions and always get them wrong? Do you question who you should be in a relationship with, or when to start doing something, or which jobs to apply for, or which task to do first? Forcing your brain out of emotional mode and into analytical mode can be the solution you need to help move you forward.

☑ For Team Indecisive: Inventory Your Past Decisions

First, you want to figure out all the instances in which you've previously had to make a decision similar to the one you are facing. For example, jobs you've taken, money you've spent, or experiences you've participated in. Go back as far as you can and write them all down. Then write the result of each decision. When you look at the results, did many—or most—of these decisions turn out okay? Any of them? It's likely you make good decisions more often than you think—it's just that the one or two negative results and experiences are much more memorable (remember: "If it bleeds, it leads") and may have caused all the positive instances to disappear from your memory. Doing an inventory like this helps to show you that you're likely better at decision-making than you might believe.

Jessica—Dating Data

When Jessica and her husband first started dating, she was completely paralyzed with doubt about whether he was "right" for her. Because she was thirty-four and "still" single, she felt all her previous relationships had been disastrous and she had no confidence in her ability to make a good choice about this relationship. She was unable to trust her own judgment, and she broke up with him not once but twice in the first six months they were dating.

For Jessica to gain perspective, we asked her to make a list of past boyfriends since her first year at college and then to rate them on a scale between "Amazing People I Could Have Potentially Married" to "Disastrous Situations with Someone Who Would Have Likely Destroyed My Entire Life."

After writing down the name of each boyfriend and considering the facts around each relationship, Jessica had eleven names on the list, and only two of them qualified as "disastrous." And one of those two was immediately after a breakup and was an obvious rebound! It turns out that nine of her boyfriends had been wonderful human beings. That's an 82 percent success rate! (Jessica realized it may have been the best grade she ever received in her life.) She discovered that she had better judgment than she gave herself credit for (the fact that she broke up with all of them was more about her commitment issues, which is a completely different topic!). Writing out the facts about the people she had chosen to be with and seeing the list in black and white gave her the confidence in herself that she needed to move forward in her current relationship . . . and although it's not easy, she's managed to stay happily married for many years.

We all make judgment errors in our lives, but our ADHD brains seem to hold on to the negative much more strongly than the positive, making us believe that we don't know what's best for us, when in fact, we usually do.

☑ For Team Impulsive: Stay in Analytical Mode

When you base your decisions on facts rather than restlessness, frustration, impatience, or other emotions, you'll usually make better choices.

Questions to ask yourself include:

- Is this the best way to make the result I want happen, or is this just a feel-better Band-Aid for now?
- What's the potential impact if I get it wrong?
- Is it something I can change if I regret my choice later?
- How much will it hold other things up if I wait to decide?

WHAT'S YOUR OVERARCHING THEME?

This is one of my all-time favorites. Decision-making can be simplified when you identify what you *ultimately* really need and want in your life. Putting a name on what it is—whether it's calm, stability, ease, fun, love, health, freedom, patience, money, or family—lets you zero in on what's important by using that word to help guide your decisions. Think of it as choosing a "theme" for your week, the month, the year, or your life!

☑ What one word would you use to sum up what you ultimately want? Write your word on a piece of paper or sticky note and place it where you will see it often throughout the day to keep it front and center.

When I did this for myself years ago, I thought about what I really wanted and needed in my life at the time, and to my surprise, I chose the word *ease*. By having the word *ease* as my focal point when making decisions, I would ask myself, *Does this choice lead to more ease or less ease?* It honestly simplified almost every choice I was faced with. I was shocked at how many seemingly logical choices I almost made that would have taken me directly to a path of stress, excitement, overwhelm, and stimulus . . . basically everything I was used to, and the exact opposite of what I ultimately wanted.

Over the years, basing decisions on a single theme has proven to be a valuable tool not only for me but for many others. If your theme resonates with you deeply, you should also write it in your notebook to remind yourself of it years from now.

☑ Correct and Continue

If fear of making a mistake is what prevents you from committing to a choice, you're not alone. Many people put off decisions just to make sure we don't mess up anything (or everything). We forget the wisdom we learned in kindergarten: everybody makes mistakes. Everybody! Scientists, CEOs, doctors, judges, parents, professional athletes, teachers, inventors, spiritual leaders, you, me, *everybody*. Think about it—nobody (except NASA) knows exactly how many course corrections the Apollo 11 mission made on its journey, but we do know that *nobody cares*, because it ultimately brought the first humans to the moon!

Even if you put a lot of pressure on yourself to make the "right" decision every time, it's easier to take the first step when you realize that you can almost always course-correct potential "mistakes" along the way and choose again.

Ask yourself any or all of these questions:

- If I weren't afraid of making a mistake, what would I choose?
- If I make the "wrong" choice, will I or other people be okay?
- Is this choice irreversible, or will there be a chance to choose again?

Paige—Stuck in Unknowns

Paige often finds herself paralyzed with indecision. She is a loving single mom of three children, and ever since her divorce, she's been incredibly overwhelmed and often becomes immobilized by "analysis paralysis"—viewing all decisions as not only important but permanent. It's all or nothing, all the time. She blames herself for her divorce and has a huge fear of making other mistakes, even if it's an inconsequential choice about where to hang her art in the apartment she moved into almost a year ago.

Never knowing what to do when, she felt completely disorganized in every area of her life. She was behind at work, wasn't taking care of herself, her apartment was a mess, and she wasn't spending quality time with her kids the way she wanted to. Paige's inability to make even small decisions was essentially affecting everything she could think of—time with family, her health, her career, making her home comfortable, and more.

To help Paige learn to make decisions more easily again, we started by having her choose one decision-making area (for now) that seemed the simplest for her to take on—to feel better by exercising more—and then had her break down the process toward that goal into incremental steps. She chose a gym in her area by limiting herself to only three options, took a trial fitness class, then signed up for two more classes, entering them into her calendar with action words in bold and all caps to visually reinforce her commitment and make it harder to back out. Ultimately, she enrolled in regular weekly classes. Her success in making choices with regular exercise built her confidence for when she faced other decisions in her life.

We also helped Paige see that she didn't need to live with every choice forever. Things that were driving her crazy, like choosing what art to hang on her walls, could be revisited. We had her see that she could, in fact, correct and continue, and in six months, if she wants to change things around, she can because she's actually not legally married to any of it! We went so far as to have her write a sticky note that said, "I'm allowed to change this piece of art in the next six months," and stick it on the corner of the frame before hanging it.

Taking away the permanence of most of her decisions and making them happen step-by-step helped her to move forward the way she needed to. (PS: After a few weeks she threw away the sticky note—she didn't need it anymore.)

Paige has now adopted the mantra "Your best decision is your best guess with the information you have at the time." Getting unstuck from indecision has freed up time for her to spend with her children, have a healthy exercise routine, and feel more in control of how, where, and with whom she spends her time.

HOW DO YOU FEEL ABOUT YOU?

This is another decision-making method that I rely on frequently and resonates with a lot of women. It's 100 percent unscientific and has elicited a few eye rolls, but for me, and many others, it works—especially when faced with "What should I do, should I do this, or should I do that?" scenarios.

☑ When facing any decision, imagine that you have already made a particular choice. Next, ask yourself, *How does this choice make me feel about myself?* If you feel good about yourself for having made that choice, it's likely a good decision. If you don't feel good about yourself for having made that choice, it's likely the wrong decision for you at this time.

Here are a few recent examples from our clients: *I told my friend I'd help with a big dinner for her and her family on Sunday because she's been sick all week, but I just found out that my sister is coming to town for the day, and she invited me out for dinner on Sunday with some of our other friends. I really want to be with my sister and our friends, especially because it'll be fun, and being with my sick friend won't be that fun, and I know I can't do both since both are at the same time. I'm 95 percent leaning toward being with my sister until I ask, "How will I feel about myself?" for canceling on my friend to go out with my sister. Instantly, the decision is clear.*

Or: *I'm exhausted. Should I try to make my 8:00 a.m. workout? If I go, how would I feel about myself? If I don't go, how would I feel about myself?*

Or: *My relationship has been feeling stagnant for months. Should I call back that man I met yesterday? If I do, how will I feel about myself? If I don't, how will I feel about myself?*

Try it, and you may be surprised by what a fast and effective way it is to help you make decisions.

Whether you tend to take much too long to make decisions and then, when you finally choose, immediately second-guess yourself, or you make rash decisions and jump in with both feet without looking, you can get better at decision-making and have much less chaos in your life as a result.

Choose (!) one or two go-to strategies from this chapter for when you're faced with a decision. If you've tried something and it isn't a great fit, try something else. Keep whatever works for you and toss the rest. Correct and continue. Remember you can always choose again.

ADHD-Friendly Quick Summary

- When it comes to making decisions, ADHDers can be indecisive or impulsive—either can get in the way of achieving what you want.
- Place a limit on your decision-making: time limit, budget limit, color limit, and amount limit, and set rules to force you to press Pause if you tend to make impulsive decisions.

- Stay in analytical mode and rely on *facts* rather than emotions to drive your decision-making.
- Decide on one ultimate theme you want in your life to direct your decisions.
- Remember that when (not if) you make an incorrect choice, most times you can simply correct and continue. Onward.
- Ask how a choice makes you feel about yourself before going forward.

ONE FOCUS

Pick a Theme, Any Theme!

Whether you're indecisive or impulsive, each day for one week, try limiting your options by choosing the main theme you identified a few pages ago (calm, ease, fun, love, health . . .) on which to base your decisions. By doing this, you're forcing your brain to work in analytical mode and focus not on one small decision itself but on how it will further your ultimate goals. Once you have your theme, for every key decision you are faced with this week, ask yourself, *Does this choice lead to more* ________? That small switch will get your brain out of emotion mode and make choosing much simpler and more effective.

14

The Facts Are Friendly

Facts are extremely powerful, as they're one of the *only* things that can supersede emotion in an ADHDer's brain. *The sun will set today at 6:45 p.m.* is a fact regardless of how you feel about it. For a woman with ADHD whose emotions tend to dictate her reality or who can only see what might be wrong in any given situation, turning her laser focus on the facts can be not only grounding but blissfully liberating.

Facts are extremely powerful, as they're one of the *only* things that can supersede emotion in an ADHDer's brain.

The facts of the world are what is. The facts are reality. And the facts are friendly because they are indisputable. *I am a woman typing on my laptop. The sun is out. My dogs are sleeping. There is a water bottle, a box of tissues, six books, a hair clip, and my kid's pencil case on the table.* This is what is, right now, and I can't make any of it be different at this exact moment.

Fact: Reality is the way things are regardless of whether we like it or not. Can you think of the last time you thought something shouldn't happen but it just went right on happening anyway? You'll notice that every time there's a discrepancy between your expectations and the actual outcome, outcome wins every time.

Find the Facts!

☑ Today and tomorrow, do your best to notice the facts of the world. Whether you are at home, at school, at work, with your family, driving, or at a store, take note of what is. Avoid adding your interpretation of what you *think* is or *should* be happening. Just notice the facts, as they are, in the moment.

"My spouse is . . ."

"The weather is . . ."

"The traffic is . . ."

"My boss is . . ."

"The tree outside my window is . . ."

Stick to what you observe to be inherently true and indisputable. "My spouse shouldn't be doing that" is not a fact. "My boss is a jerk" is not a fact. "The weather sucks today" is not a fact. "My bank account should be much bigger" is not a fact. These are all opinions, wishes, and interpretations.

"My spouse is napping on the couch" is a fact. "My boss is accountable for what our team produces" is a fact. The facts can give you needed perspective by taking you out of your automatic emotional reactions and into a more objective, analytical response.

NEGATIVITY IS NOT A FACT

There may be a voice in your head that is hypercritical and spends more time recounting your "failures" than singing your praises. This negativity continually hammers your self-esteem and can taint your overall outlook on life. Luckily, focusing on the *positive* facts and just those facts is a tried-and-true way to counter much of that negative self-talk, and this approach has worked successfully for our clients time and again.

FACTS ARE FRIENDLY

Remember Your Achievements and Battle Self-Doubt

Visuals are extremely powerful to us and capture more of our attention than simply thinking about something will. Regardless of how terrible you're feeling about yourself at any moment, creating a visual of your actual factual accomplishments, both big and small, that you can look at shows without question what you have achieved, positive things you have done, and is a solid reminder of what you are absolutely capable of doing again.

Keep in mind that the facts do *not* include wishes, affirmations, strong opinions, or mind-blowing amazing ideas.

☑ Official Recipe for a Facts Are Friendly List

For this exercise, you'll need a piece of paper to make a Facts Are Friendly list, and a designated **Wall of Attention**, which is the location you'll use for posting this list. Ideally, your Wall of Attention will be someplace you already see at least a couple of times a day, every day—maybe your bathroom mirror, near your coffee maker, next to your computer, or on the fridge.

Why do you need a Wall of Attention? If your list is in your notebook or on your computer, you won't ever see it—the notebook gets closed and put on the shelf, and the computer gets shut down. Your Facts Are Friendly list needs to always be visible without your having to turn it on or look for it.

☑ 1. Take out a sheet of paper and write in big letters across the top: The FACTS Are FRIENDLY (make the word *FACTS* nice and big to catch your brain's attention) or print out the template at: adhdcoaching.com/factsarefriendly.

ADHDCOACHING.COM Date: ______

The FACTS Are FRIENDLY!

© 2020 Shanna Pearson. All rights reserved.

Take ten minutes to think about and *write down* everything that you have accomplished over the past five years, or twenty years, or three weeks, whatever time period feels right for you. The physical act of writing down your FACTUAL accomplishments is kinesthetic, and your brain will be forced to slow down just enough to internalize the information. It will also provide you with permanent visual proof of these accomplishments so you can refer to them the next time self-doubt creeps in.

2. Remember as you write down these facts, you are listing positive things that you've actually done, created in your life, and are proud of, *not* goals or positive affirmations. In addition to any of your bigger successes, you need to include smaller things, too—as many as you can! Like calling your elderly parents to check in or getting to bed before 11:00 p.m. two times this week.

   These must be facts. Indisputable. And they can include some of the following:
   * The work you do, or have done, at any point in your life that you're most proud of. Volunteer work counts.
   * The people you've positively impacted or helped in some way, big or small. Friends, family, acquaintances, colleagues, and people whose names you don't remember. Scroll through photos on your phone if it helps to ring a bell.
   * What you've stayed committed to: your health, specific friendships, your career, school, a romantic relationship, your finances, an important cause . . .
   * Accomplishments or situations where you've done something well, whether it was recognized or not.
   * Any compliments, gratitude, or praise you have received from anyone verbally, or over email or text—ever. Who was it and what did they say?

3. ***Bonus Activity*:** Write down one or two emotionally descriptive words about how it *felt* for you to accomplish each (or at least one) of the facts on your list. Focusing on the emotion you personally experienced, which will likely be a positive one, will help to elicit this feeling again when you think about these accomplishments in the future.

4. Post your Facts Are Friendly list on your Wall of Attention. This SHOWS your brain what you've accomplished and also what you can (absolutely!) achieve again, to remind yourself

how awesome you are, because your brain has a tendency to forget.

☑ 5. Update your Facts Are Friendly list, or create a new one, every six weeks (put a reminder in your calendar to make sure you do this).

☑ 6. Whenever you are feeling doubt about your ability or unsure of the value of your past accomplishments, simply look at your Facts Are Friendly list. Stand up and read the list out loud—as a declaration of the facts of your accomplishments. *If you feel like having some fun, read your facts out loud imitating someone famous or funny*. Not only will it be more memorable, speaking in a different voice or accent will slow you down as you're reading, so you won't breeze through it, allowing the information to be absorbed more deeply.

The physical act of writing down your FACTUAL accomplishments is kinesthetic, and your brain will be forced to slow down just enough to internalize the information.

If You're Having Difficulty Getting Started

Some people have a hard time coming up with *anything* for their Facts Are Friendly list at first, but trust me, that is your ADHD mind being overwhelmed. When you take a few minutes, you will realize there are plenty of wins, achievements, and positive experiences in your history.

These don't need to be monumental accomplishments; even little things count. One item for your list can be that you made it to chapter 14 of this book (unless you just randomly opened it to this page). Another could be "I got this book, and I am reading it instead of letting it sit on the shelf unopened with all my other unread books." Continue asking yourself about your recent wins, big and small, until you have three or four achievements to put on the list.

The rule is that what you write down has to be positive *facts* like "I got that job" or "I graduated from college" (even if it was thirty years ago) or "I've gotten my kid to school on time for the past four days" or "I finally sent those emails I've been putting off" or "I haven't gotten in an argument with anyone for the past two days *(or two hours)*." Facts are indisputable and are something your mind can't ever negate.

Beyond proving your own abilities to yourself, the Facts Are Friendly list can help in other ways as well:

☑ What IS Versus What IF

For women with ADHD, what-if thinking can be a way of life, especially because what-ifs are everywhere, your mind has no separate place to put them, so they remain intertwined with everything else and are incredibly engaging. The what-ifs usually dwell on every possible catastrophe, ignoring potential positive or neutral outcomes even when the imagined disaster is far less likely. When what-ifs take on a negative spin—which they usually do—they can turn everyday stressful thoughts or situations into something blown way out of proportion.

You can start to quell the catastrophic what-ifs that your brain naturally gravitates to and never wants to let go of by keeping your focus on the simple, non-negatable facts of "What Is." This is easier said than done; however, if you make it a goal to come up with five potential *positive and realistic* possibilities for each What-If scenario, you'll begin to feel less engulfed by the alarming thoughts your mind is creating.

☑ Fact-Focused Evaluation for Building Self-Trust

Similar to what Jessica did in the previous chapter when taking an inventory of her past relationships, you can challenge any of your negative beliefs about *yourself* by doing an inventory of what's gone well for you: How many times this year have you put effort into something and had it turn out close to the way you wanted? When were you on time this week? What was a good decision you made this month? Name the people you've had a good experience with this week.

You can challenge any of your negative beliefs about *yourself* by doing an inventory.

When you perform a fact-focused evaluation, you quickly shift out of the emotional and into the analytical. This allows your brain to recognize your legitimate accomplishments.

☑ The Daily Facts Are Friendly: For When You Feel Like You Never Get Enough Done

Many of us feel that no matter how fast we're moving, how much we're doing, or how stressed out we are trying to stay on top of everything, it's never enough. With poor time awareness, something you did hours ago can seem like it happened so long ago that it feels like you did it last week—when it was today. This technique will help you take note of what you've factually done—both big and small.

At the end of the day, open your notebook, write the date, set a timer for two minutes, and write down everything you accomplished that day—no matter how minor it may seem. Aim to have at least ten things on your list. Eating a healthy-ish snack can be one. If you sent that email or text, or made that phone call, write it down. If you remembered to hug someone goodbye for the day, write it down. If you put something away that you've been ignoring for a while, write it down. If you made *any* progress on a project or learned something new, or if you made someone else feel good, write it down. If you managed to exercise, write that down, and if you pushed yourself more than usual when you were exercising, write that down, too.

The idea is that while we can feel as if we are getting absolutely nothing done or are spinning our wheels going nowhere, there are actually a multitude of small wins each day. Becoming aware of these moments will reinforce how competent you are and how much more you're capable of. Give yourself kudos for all of it, too!

It's easy to get totally caught up in our current nonstop swirl of emotions and thoughts, but when you focus on the positive facts about your life and situations—those pieces of information that your ADHD brain often overlooks—and notice what you're honestly capable of and what actually is true, it'll be much easier for you to believe in *yourself*, and know that you can accomplish equally good things in the future.

ADHD-Friendly Quick Summary

- Facts Are Friendly is essential for battling self-doubt and negative self-talk.
- Facts are one of the *only* things that override emotion in an ADHDer's brain.
- Create a Facts Are Friendly list to remind yourself of the positives behind what you've actually done and are doing, big and small. Keep it where you'll see it every day.
- Focus on the emotion of how each factual accomplishment felt.
- Your Facts Are Friendly list *cannot* include affirmations, wishes, or goals. Only indisputable facts.
- "What Is" is fact. What-ifs are often based on fear and are not factual.
- Use a fact-based inventory when you have difficulty trusting your decisions.
- If you feel like you never get enough done, do a daily Facts Are Friendly.

ONE FOCUS

Create Your First Facts Are Friendly List

1. Print out the template at *adhdcoaching.com/factsarefriendly* or take out a piece of paper and at the top write in large letters: The FACTS Are FRIENDLY.
2. Write out five to ten of your actual, factual accomplishments—big or small. These are positive things you have done or created in your life, things you are proud of, and so on.
3. Write down one or two descriptive words about how each point impacted you emotionally or how it felt to accomplish it.
4. Post your Facts Are Friendly list on your Wall of Attention at eye level for you to see the visual non-negatable facts of what you've been capable of doing!

When you first start to use your Facts Are Friendly list, you'll notice, at the very least, how quickly it interrupts and distracts you from your negative thoughts. As you keep updating your successes, you'll start to notice a shift where these facts gradually replace negativity. Over time, this habit not only boosts your confidence but also nurtures a mindset that embraces achievement and keeps your motivation alive and thriving.

15

Create Juicy Goals

How many of us have something we want to achieve but find that our days are filled with doing just about everything else *except* the things that will help us achieve it? If that's you, you're in excellent company. *The #1 reason a person with ADHD does not achieve the results they want is because their focus—what they're paying attention to and actually doing—is not in alignment with their goals!*

Having goals gives our minds focus and direction—two things most of us with ADHD could use a bit more of. This chapter will give you strategies for creating bigger and juicier goals that will motivate you and keep you in the game. It will also help you to discover the *why* behind your goals that will not only clarify them but give you the motivation to pursue them—and be excited about it!

GOING FOR THE GOAL OR GOING THROUGH THE MOTIONS?

If you really want to go somewhere but have no idea where it is, it'll be difficult to get there. Imagine you have a GPS and you've just entered a destination, except you don't turn when it tells you to turn, or you only focus on part of the directions. You're unlikely to get where you want to go easily or at all. It's the same for the goals you set for yourself. When you focus on the wrong things, go off course, or get distracted from your goals, you will not reach your destination, which is extremely frustrating!

The #1 reason a person with ADHD does not achieve the results they want is because their focus—what they're paying attention to and actually doing—is not in alignment with their goals!

☑ So, before we jump in further, let's do this two-minute exercise to ascertain where you stand with your own goals. In your notebook, write your responses to the following:

1. **What is one goal you have?**
2. **What actions have you been taking regularly to achieve that goal?**

Whatever you wrote will be a giant clue as to why you are on your way to reaching your goal, or why you aren't (especially if you didn't have any actions to write down).

A lot of people with ADHD live in survival mode, just trying to get through the day, which makes creating meaningful goals seem impossible—especially when your most pressing need is to get out the door on time without having to run back inside three times because you forgot something. Just like right now as you're reading this, you might be interested in identifying what your bigger goals are but at the same time you want to put it off for later because you know you have to start figuring out what to make for dinner soon.

Furthermore, you may not even think about setting goals for yourself because:

- You doubt you can pull it off.
- You think it will require too much work.
- You feel like the thing you want is off-limits to you.
- You have absolutely no idea *how* to pursue that goal.

- You're already stretched so thin with endless things on your plate, it feels impossible to think about *anything*, let alone a new goal.

Thankfully, there are strategies to counter those self-doubts and other obstacles, to help get you on the road to choosing and, more importantly, achieving your goals.

☑ CHOOSE YOUR FOCUS

While we all have a hundred things we need to juggle throughout the day, we also have lots of great ideas running around in our heads. Ideas are important, but they're limitless. Many brilliant people die with lots of brilliant ideas that they never made happen, so a goal needs to be much more than an idea.

Here are some pointers for choosing a meaningful goal to focus on so it can have your time and energy:

- Be sure the goal is YOURS—not your spouse's, mother's, sibling's, or best friend's—it should be yours and yours alone.
- What will the impact of this goal be? Choose a goal that will make a meaningful difference to you (not just another to-do task item).
- What pain will occur if you do not achieve the goal? This should also be significant.

It's possible that you can't think of a particularly fulfilling goal that comes to mind right now, and if that's the case, here are a few suggestions to get you started.

- Make a "want" list of three items in order of importance. It will be easier to come up with three items rather than just one because of how overwhelming it can be for ADHDers to choose only one—of anything! You can alleviate the difficulty of choosing just one by narrowing your options to three. This will make it much easier to identify which is truly your most compelling goal.

- Think about what you wanted when you were younger. At ten? Fifteen? Twenty-five? Do any aspects of those wishes and desires resonate with you today?
- Who is someone you admire and why? What is it about them? What do they do? Does anything about them inspire something you want to strive for?
- Choose a goal based on how you'd like to *feel*. Even if you don't know exactly what you want to do or have, you likely know how you want to feel.

Alleviate the difficulty of choosing just one by narrowing your options to three.

☑ MAKE IT EMOTIONAL

Because people with ADHD are driven by their emotions, you are compelled to seek out what is interesting and exciting. So when you have aspirations or goals, they absolutely need to be connected to your emotions to make them achievable. If you're less emotionally engaged, your brain's need for stimulus will often take you off course—consciously or unconsciously. But you can use your need for stimulus to your advantage! As you've likely experienced, stimulus can be negative (taking you further away from your goals) or it can be positive (bringing you closer to your goals). Examples of positive stimuli are feelings of excitement, deep fulfillment, and anticipation.

The trick is to work with your brain's need for stimulus to make your goals as powerful as they can be! It's much harder to quit our goals when they resonate deeply with us, especially when there is a nice Big Why behind them.

Work with your brain's need for stimulus to make your goals as powerful as they can be!

The BIG Why

If you've ever had a four-year-old in your life, you know that they ask "Why?" about basically Every. Single. Thing. They also don't accept the first answer they get but will go further into each "Why?" I'm going to ask you to bring the same attitude to your goals and dreams.

Your Big Why is a big deal. A Big Why is what your soul wants. It is more meaningful, naturally motivating, and powerful enough not to be taken out by random distractions. It taps into your deeper motivation, and your goals will never be juicy without it. If you have ADHD, you shouldn't even consider having a big goal that doesn't include a Big Why. We tend to take action based on our emotions, so the more personal and heart-filling you can make your Big Why for any goal, the easier it will be to reach it. Or, as we say: *The bigger the why, the easier the how.*

If you have ADHD, you shouldn't even consider having a big goal that doesn't include a Big Why.

The Big Why fueling your goal should be something more powerful than "I want that" or "I really should do that." It should have an emotional charge that makes it invigorating and genuinely holds your attention.

☑ With any goal that you have (you can think of one now) ask yourself: *Why* do you want that? *Why* should you really do that? What is the *deeper* reason you want it? *Why?* Keep asking why until you hit a response that lights you up—it may take asking *why* at least five times to get there. Maybe your goal is really about freedom, creating more joy and happiness, leaving a small mark in the world, creating something meaningful for your family—anything that truly gets you excited.

Cynthia—Using Her Big Why

Cynthia is a wife and the mother of four children. She is pulled in a lot of directions, struggles with balance in her home and church life, and frequently feels like she comes up short. She often feels overwhelmed and disorganized, which she thought contributed to how unbelievably messy her home was. Because of the constant mess, she wasn't comfortable hosting the women in her church community. With four kids, Cynthia has a lot going on, and the idea of setting goals for anything she might want felt completely impossible.

When Cynthia's oldest turned fifteen, she realized that her kids, who were the most important thing in her life, were growing up and wouldn't be living with her forever!

We helped Cynthia formulate a specific, emotionally charged, juicy goal: to spend much more time with her children, which was backed up by a powerful Big Why: because they would be moving out within a few years (so soon!) and she might never have another chance to be fully present in their lives like she does right now.

We connected her other goals, like having a tidier home, to her Juicy Goal of spending more time with her kids. Before, she was too disorganized and didn't have time to just clean the house, but now she was driven to "clean the house so that I can invite my friends and my kids' friends over to a home that is inviting and welcoming for guests, and where it'll feel nicer for our family to spend time together."

To make it happen, we set up a schedule so each child helped with some aspect of cleaning or organizing each day, and the children were in charge of choosing the music they listened to when it was their turn. Afterward, they did something fun together like watch a show, bake something simple, or play a game. Not only did she get to spend much more time with her kids, but she finally felt excited about the prospect of being the home where kids wanted to gather. Her Big Why allowed her to connect and stick to her goal and cut through the overwhelm to give her time, attention, and energy to what she most wanted in her life.

☑ Make Your Goals Juicier!

Here are a few examples of how to transform average goals into Juicy Goals that will make you want to get out of bed every morning without hitting Snooze. You'll notice there's an easy formula for this:

1. Make your goal more specific, and
2. Attach a Big Why.

Change "I want to make more money" (sure, who doesn't?) into "I want to triple my savings by next year." *Why?* "So I can have enough savings to feel financially secure, alleviate my constant anxiety about money, and finally be able to consider buying a small cabin in the woods where I can escape to every summer."

Change "I want to get in shape" (heard that one a million times) into "I want to be able to walk five miles a day by February 1." *Why?* "So I can hike the Pacific Crest Trail next summer with my friends without passing out or seriously embarrassing myself."

See how these goals get *much* more interesting when you identify the personal reasons behind them? Always do your best to keep what you want front and center. When a Big Why isn't big enough or a goal isn't juicy enough, any earthly distraction can take you off track, and you won't have the motivation you need to follow through on them. The more specific your Juicy Goal is, backed up by a deeply meaningful Big Why, the more impossible it will be for your brain to ignore.

Yina—Reconnecting with Herself

Yina was diagnosed with ADHD ten years ago and is now in her early forties. She has many goals, but most are driven by her thinking about what she is "supposed to have" and "supposed to do" rather than things that have personal meaning for her. She sought my help because she had been feeling more distracted than usual and recently had been waking up every morning feeling miserable and didn't know why. She is very supportive of her family and friends and is always available for them, but then she doesn't show up for herself and barely acknowledges what she wants, since she's always felt that she wants so many different things!

Yina had reached a senior manager position many years ago, but it's been difficult for her to advance further in her job, and she feels completely trapped. Outside her job, she has dozens of creative and meaningful ideas that involve fashion, architecture, and real estate—including dreaming of owning her own home one day where she can flex her creativity with interior design, create a dream kitchen, make a great space for entertaining, and feel independent! The trouble is that Yina is so entrenched in her current story—manager, dutiful wife, good daughter, sacrificing friend—that she can't allow herself to believe in another story, one that prioritizes her own desires.

In the past, she's been able to achieve certain goals in some areas of her life (career) but then got completely sidetracked from her creative pursuits. When Yina began to focus on her Big Why, she was able to take a chance on putting her own dreams into action. She focused on what the goal of owning her own home would bring to her life. We then created a plan to achieve her most meaningful goal and worked on it one step at a time. Now as she approaches what once seemed like an impossible dream, she wakes up happier and more confident because she feels herself moving toward achieving what she truly wants—for herself.

☑ "So That I Can"

Your brain wants—*it needs*—to be motivated by something that matters to you. Reframing your goals, and the steps you need to take to achieve them, to clarify what you will gain personally and adding the words *so that I can,* will help to connect your ultimate goal with the action you are undertaking. Working out three times a week isn't torture when you add, *so that I can feel better, sleep better, look better, and be stronger!* Going to that social event for work when you *never* go to those events isn't a nightmare when you see it as an opportunity to potentially address the social anxiety you've been trying to manage for most of your adult life.

This simple shift in perspective can help transform something that is practical into something that is exciting. Women with ADHD will especially benefit from taking advantage of the emotional connection between the heart and the mind. When the two are in alignment, the impact is powerful. Reframing your goals to be more engaging and "juicier" will allow you to stay focused. You can clean up your house or apartment because it needs to be done (ugh!), or you can picture your space as your personal retreat and see how cleaning it doesn't only enhance your daily living experience but can also infuse some much-needed tranquility into your life.

WHEN YOU HAVE TOO MANY GOALS

While some women with ADHD may have trouble coming up with one goal to reach for, other women have a more complicated problem—there are too many things they would like to accomplish! If this resonates with you, you can make reaching your goals possible by deciding which are *most* significant for you. Which of your goals, if any, have a Big Why attached to them, versus which are just "interesting" or high-stimulus sidetracks that aren't deeply meaningful to you in the long run? You can make a list of all your many goals right now, then go down the list, cross off the ones that *might* be sidetracks, and highlight the one or two goals that have the biggest why behind them.

Pamela—Too Many Goals

Pamela is a creative marketing professional in her fifties. She is a big thinker with an endless stream of ideas, and they all become major goals—conferences she could produce, new business ideas, new products, books she wants to write—she even puts time into creating outlines for them. She wants to do them all, right now, yet she can never start anything. She'll be interested in one, move on to the next and the next, and then become so overwhelmed because of all the ideas and the directions they can take her that she doesn't pursue any of them and feels like a failure because of it.

When Pamela came for help, she was feeling totally depleted and defeated. She said that deep down she didn't trust herself to take on any of the projects she comes up with, because she believed that because she had ADHD, she was destined to be disorganized and scattered—traits she worked very hard to disguise at work. She also believed she wouldn't be able to follow through on anything anyway.

Our first step for Pamela was to slow down and focus on her Big Why. She soon realized that generating all her amazing ideas was her brain seeking stimulation and helping her stay one foot out the door just in case her job didn't work out.

After further careful examination, she realized, to her surprise, that what she truly wanted was to excel at her current job! The job she had been in for the past three years already gave her so much of what she wanted. She loved the projects, the pay, her coworkers, the clients she was helping; yet she hadn't been able to see any of this, because her mind had been distracted by all her other exciting ideas.

Her fulfillment was right in her own backyard. Realizing this allowed her to become emotionally engaged by her job and focus more on her current responsibilities. We also implemented a dedicated notebook to park the ideas for all her new initiatives for a time when, and if, she wants to pursue them in the future.

HOW TO ACHIEVE YOUR GOALS

A goal can be something simple (*Clear out my inbox*), or it can be an attempt to fulfill a major childhood dream (*Open my own dance studio*). If you think about your goal as the ultimate destination that you plug into your GPS, some of these steps are the turns and directions that will take you there.

☑ Write the answers to the following in your notebook to help clarify where you want to go.

1. What exactly is your goal? (Example: *I want to spend more quality time with my partner.*)
2. What's the Big Why behind your goal that makes it important for you? Remember, for ADHDers, the emotional impact is what will keep you motivated and moving forward. (*Because when "we" are connected and happy, everything and everyone in our lives, including our kids, are happier.*) Double-check that you are emotionally connected to your goal. Ask yourself what will happen if you *never* achieve this goal. Is that something you're okay with?
3. How can you make this goal more specific or measurable? For example:

   ***What*:** Date nights that are fun and interesting; uplifting conversations that stay away from all my work-related complaints.

   ***How Many*:** Two fun date nights per month; one uplifting, complaint-free conversation per week.

   ***When*:** Date night every second Thursday, and at least one intentional conversation every weekend.

These specifics will help you to break your goal into mini goals to take it from "I would really like to______" to actually accomplishing it!

4. Keep it visible! A key to keeping that Juicy Goal front and center in your mind (and where your mind goes, your attention and energy will follow) is to write it out on a piece of paper and put it where you will see it multiple times throughout the day. In the previous chapter, you wrote your Facts Are Friendly list and posted it somewhere visible on your Wall of Attention (whether it's a wall or not). Your current goal, along with your Big Why, can be posted there as well.

☑ Make It More ADHD-Friendly

1. If your goal is large: Divide it into five to ten small simple steps and write them down. Next, break each step into smaller steps, if possible, so you can complete them easily. Write these smaller steps down to embed them deeper in your mind and to serve as a checklist.
2. Prioritize and sequence the items so that you can follow the "order of operations" *exactly like a recipe*. (More on this in the next chapter.)
3. Set a deadline or completion date. Be definitive. Don't say, "Next week." Say, "By next Tuesday at noon."
4. Make it real: Take out your calendar (right now) and schedule the specific steps into your week at the times when you know you'll be able to do them to reach your deadline.

A goal by itself is only an item on your wish list and is super easy for your stimulus-seeking—and often overwhelmed—brain to ignore. When you have a Juicy Goal fueled by a Big Why, you will have something to move toward that is connected to a deeper part of your essence and taps into your emotions *so that you can* eventually achieve everything that's meaningful to you.

ADHD-Friendly Quick Summary

- The primary reason you don't achieve your goals is because your immediate focus—what you're doing and paying attention to—is not in alignment with what you actually want.
- Choose your goals based on what's meaningful to you, rather than task items.
- If you don't have goals or don't know *what* you want, create a goal based on how you want to *feel*.
- A Juicy Goal attached to a Big Why generates the emotional stimulus you need to stay engaged and on track.
- *"The Bigger the Why, the Easier the How."* The clearer and more meaningful your Big Why behind your goal is, the better the chance you have of achieving it.
- If your small goals aren't feeling meaningful, add in *"so that I can"* to increase the energy and personal significance behind them.
- If you have too many goals, narrow them down and figure out which are more closely connected to your Big Why.
- Make sure your goals have specific and measurable small action steps so you know when and how to move forward, and easily measure your progress.

ONE FOCUS

Get in Touch with Your Big Why

1. Choose one goal that you are working toward, or that you would like to work on, and write it down.
2. Ask yourself *why* you want to achieve that goal. Ask why again. And again. You can ask yourself up to ten times if you need to and go as many levels deep as it takes to reach a Big Why that really resonates with your soul.
3. Write down your Big Why.
4. Write down one tiny step you can take *each day* this week toward your goal.

If you're up for it, post your Juicy Goal and your Big Why on your Wall of Attention to keep it front of mind. At the end of one week, check in with yourself to see how you've already started moving closer to your goal.

16

Overcome Your Overwhelm and Get Stuff Done

While we now know that physical hyperactivity *isn't* standard for all people with ADHD, living in a constant state of overwhelm *is* something almost every woman with ADHD struggles with. Your brain's struggle to compartmentalize means that every thought in your incredible mind feels like it has equal weight and importance. With *everything* fighting for your focus, it's difficult to determine what you need to pay attention to at any given time. This leads to feeling paralyzed by overwhelm, which then causes you to become easily distracted, impatient, impulsive, disorganized, and less able to manage your time effectively. (Sound familiar?)

While anyone can be pulled in multiple directions at once—*I have to be at work, my friend needs help, I need to get groceries, a project is due*—and we all juggle multiple responsibilities, people who have ADHD can feel overwhelmed every moment of every day!

Feeling paralyzed by overwhelm causes you to become easily distracted, impatient, impulsive, disorganized, and less able to manage your time effectively.

OVERWHELMED AND UNDERACHIEVING

Feeling overwhelmed is such a prevalent reality for us that in essence, a huge part of ADHD management *is* overwhelm management. Ironically, many people with ADHD tend to create even more overwhelm through our need for more stimulus. It's a bit of a catch-22. Your ADHD brain tries to escape overwhelm by seeking distractions in whatever grabs your attention, like gaming, chatting, snacking, online shopping, binge watching, and so on, thus jumping out of one emotion into another, seemingly more enjoyable one. The enjoyable distraction creates a temporary dopamine hit, but the fact of the matter is that you're doing something unnecessary that doesn't move you toward your goals and might even be moving you farther away from them. Maybe you spent money you didn't have or you're upset that you spent half the day mindlessly shopping for things you'll never need. Ultimately, you don't feel any better, the overwhelm grows, and you become frozen—again.

A way to visualize what overwhelm is like is to picture your moods and thoughts as being tangled together like a huge ball of multiple strands of colored yarn. It's hard to tell where one strand begins and another ends. The tangled mess is everything that is happening right now. It seems impossible to separate out your thoughts and feelings and determine the appropriate actions to take in response to each individual issue. As a result, you become even more overwhelmed, completely frozen, don't know how or where to begin, and ultimately get very little done.

Fortunately, there are ways that you can slow things down just enough to be able to untangle that ball of yarn into separate individual strands so that you're able to see which *one* thing you need to start moving forward on and then deal with each of them step by step.

BREAK IT DOWN TO GET IT DONE!

When faced with any task, most of us think about the result we want and then immediately think about all the work it will take to get there. If the task is big, this can be overwhelming to say the least. So, rather than becoming immobilized by the enormity of the process, it helps to shift your focus to the smaller steps required to get you there.

☑ Minuscule Morsels

The key word here is *minuscule*. You may have heard about "chunking things down," but for many women with ADHD, we need to think in terms of the truly microscopic. In the previous chapter about setting goals, we touched on breaking your overarching goal into small steps and then making each step even smaller by further breaking them down into tasks so small you're almost guaranteed to get them done. (And this process can—and should—also be applied to tasks that are not that fun or even remotely juicy!)

☑ A Recipe for Separation

Another way to tackle a large task or goal is to think of it like following a recipe. If you want to cook or bake something, you work through each step, one at a time, usually in a particular order, to get the results you want. Imagine you promised to make a homemade apple pie for someone's birthday and you've never made one before. The idea of doing this might be overwhelming. However, if the very first step was simply for you to write down the ingredients you need, that would seem manageable. But if that still seems overwhelming to you (don't worry, you're not alone here!), perhaps your first tiny steps would be to find a recipe or reach out to the person whose recipe you love, and *then* write down the ingredients you need. The next step might then be to go to the store to buy the ingredients, but for some of us, that needs to be broken down further: get your keys, get out the door, and then go to the store to buy the apples and other ingredients. Once you're back in your kitchen, the next step might be to preheat your oven—something you've likely done before, so it's easy to do. Then you'll be able to tackle the actual apple pie recipe step-by-step and end up with a great dessert.

The recipe idea works the same way out of the kitchen. Let's say you have a major project to finish and you have no idea how to start. First step: gather all the ingredients you need. You might, for example, only need one ingredient, your computer, and maybe a quiet place to work—or noise-canceling headphones if you don't have a quiet spot. But if you have any other materials you need, gather them all together in one space. Then break down the task and walk through each step as if you were cooking up something in your kitchen.

Step 1: Open your laptop.

Step 2: Open the document for your project! This step is obvious, but you'd be amazed at how many of us don't ever get to step 2 because we become overwhelmed simply by *thinking* about the project, and to escape the overwhelm, we go to our social media feeds or other online distractions and end up staying there for hours.

So, without thinking about the whole project, open the document.

Step 3: Begin tackling it by *starting* with an intention of only working for thirty seconds. Or for one sentence. In other words: start.

Step 4: Stay on the project or document and continue working on any part of it for ten minutes. Set a timer. At the end of those ten minutes, without taking a break, simply aim to do five or ten more minutes. You get the idea.

If you focus on the tiny step of finding and opening a specific document, it's more likely to happen than if you're focused on tackling the entire project, which is so overwhelming that you won't know how to start and automatically jump headfirst into the next closest distraction.

SHRINKING YOUR TO-DO LIST

Most of us feel overwhelmed just by looking at the million things on our to-do lists, so we either ignore all of them, do the things that are the least important, or throw the entire list out and start working on completely new to-do items we just thought of as a sidetrack to avoid trying to figure out what to do first . . . or second . . . or . . .

Here's how you can begin to narrow your focus and get stuff done:

☑ Keep It to Three and You're Free

A lot of our clients start off with to-do lists that are over forty items long, which in itself is overwhelming. One simple way to quell the visual overwhelm is to simply use a separate *short* written list. You don't have to worry about the priority level of what's on this list—yet!

Each morning, write out a list that is uncomfortably short—just three items maximum. Tackle only the first item, and when it's completed, go to the next, bearing in mind that you're only allowed to select from the items *already* on your short list. Only when you have completed your list can you add more items. Put a check mark next to each item as you complete it so you can end the day with accomplishments rather than resignation about not getting enough done. This creates a *visual* boundary around the number of tasks you're allowing yourself to think about—and see—at any one time, helping you to feel less overwhelmed and get more done than you might imagine. Now we can start thinking about prioritizing!

☑ Prioritize and Single Handle Until Complete

Because thinking about too many things at once usually leaves ADHDers somewhat immobilized, ultimately it's best to narrow your focus to tackle just your top priority items, one at a time. This doesn't mean that the other things won't get done, just that they can be set aside for a bit. But how does an ADHDer living in an "everything all at once right now" reality begin to prioritize?

You can start by looking at your original to-do list and then writing out only the tasks that you think you need to do sooner rather than later. Keep in mind that all your tasks are already on the original list, so you know that nothing will be forgotten. For now, choose just one or two that you need to do first. You may be thinking, *Are you kidding me? There's no way I can narrow down a list of forty-six to just one or two!*

You can do it by asking yourself three magic questions—they'll apply to every item on your list:

The Three Magic Questions of Prioritization

- Which of these items has the closest deadline? Pick four or five and highlight them.
- Out of those, which has the greatest impact on your life? *Does it seriously affect my life in a major way, or just how I feel right now?* Cross out any that you are simply responding to impulsively or emotionally.
- Will there be major (negative) consequences if these don't get done today? For any to which the answer is no, move them to the back of the line. Only the highlighted tasks that remain should be on your short list.

When you write down your answers (as opposed to thinking about your responses and having them all swirling in your head), you'll see that your list will be much shorter *and* more prioritized so you can determine what to focus on today.

After asking these questions, some clients end up with zero items remaining on their list! Which, if nothing else, alleviates their stress and overwhelm since they know that while these things need to get done eventually, the world won't come crashing down if they don't *all* get done right now.

One Focus . . . Total Success

With a small, prioritized list, it's like that huge ball of yarn we mentioned earlier is reduced to three strands of different-colored yarn—each easy to see and separate from one another so you can focus on one at a time. Concentrating on one action item or problem at a time is likely the opposite of what you normally do (trying to work or focus on a hundred things at once). If you worry about limiting yourself to only one thing when *everything* is really important, know that focusing on one thing at a time will get the results you want *faster* than what you've been doing up until now. On a personal note, this was so meaningful and effective for me in my own life that "One Focus Total Success Inc." was the original name for my ADHD coaching company.

Focusing on one thing at a time will get the results you want *faster* than what you've been doing up until now.

Remember *The Karate Kid*? Instead of teaching Daniel all the basic karate moves at once, Mr. Miyagi teaches him only one simple movement to master, "wax on, wax off," and gives him a long row of cars to wax, one at a time, in a very specific way. Daniel reluctantly had to focus on "wax on, right hand, wax off, left hand," car after car. Repeating just that one circular motion over and over allowed him to master it quickly so he could move on to the next step and eventually become a karate champion. It's amazing how many of us "already know" this concept in theory, yet rarely take the time to apply it to our own lives.

Attacking one and only one thing at a time will help your brain to simplify, let you accomplish what you need to do, and do a fantastic job of protecting you from overwhelm.

CREATING SEPARATION IN TIME AND SPACE

Once upon a time during the COVID-19 pandemic, when shelter-in-place orders were being enforced and the entire world was overwhelmed, we learned from *all* our ADHD clients—who suddenly had to start working from home with a million other distractions around them (including sharing space with family members also in school and at work, causing everyone to be totally frozen and unable to get anything done)—which overwhelm management strategies genuinely worked the best for their ADHD brains! If these concepts worked under those extreme circumstances, they'll likely work for you now.

It came as little surprise that the most effective strategies involved learning to create separations in how you use your time as well as your space, to compensate for your brain's challenges with compartmentalizing.

Separation of Time

It's very common for us to believe that everything we need to do must be addressed immediately. If you don't do it *right now,* you'll simply forget to do it entirely. In truth, many of these things are not that critical and can, in fact, pull you away from your bigger goals or priorities. It's possible, even likely, that the urgency you feel is purely emotional and not at all based in fact.

☑ Now and Not Now

To override this emotional response and help you decide what to do first, separate your tasks into two categories. Create two columns, with the headings "Now" and "Not Now," and enter each to-do in the appropriate column. Then you can address only the Now items, *one at a time,* and once you are done with those, move on to the Not Now tasks.

If you're someone who tends to put everything in the Not Now category and always postpones tasks—even the things that really do need your attention immediately—sort the Not Now items by which should get done before the others, put the top ones in the Now column, and then take only the first tiny step to start working on them.

☑ Break It into Boxes

Another way to help with our overwhelm and our "everything all at once right now" reality is to create a visual representation of boxes that represent distinct separations between your daily activities. The goal of this exercise is to clarify both focused time and free time. You'll draw a box on a sheet of paper or in your notebook that visually represents a part of your day: like your morning routine, your work or school hours, family time, relationship time, and so on. Each part of your day is in its own separate box with its own activities, *including designated flex time*. In other words, you're building compartments and separations where none existed. It's helpful to imagine that each box is built with heavy impenetrable steel walls, and to draw your boxes with thick lines.

You're building compartments and separations where none existed.

Laying the hours of your day out in this way will help you to not only see but understand that even if you have a hundred things to do, you also have designated flexible time to spend on *anything* you want. Creating a visual that shows separations where none currently exist will help you create the mental space to focus on one particular task and not try to juggle or think about everything all at once.

Try this yourself:
On a sheet of paper, create one box with very thick walls for one part of your day—Morning, Afternoon, Evening—or however you want to break up your day. Below is an example of how our client Eliza created her morning box.

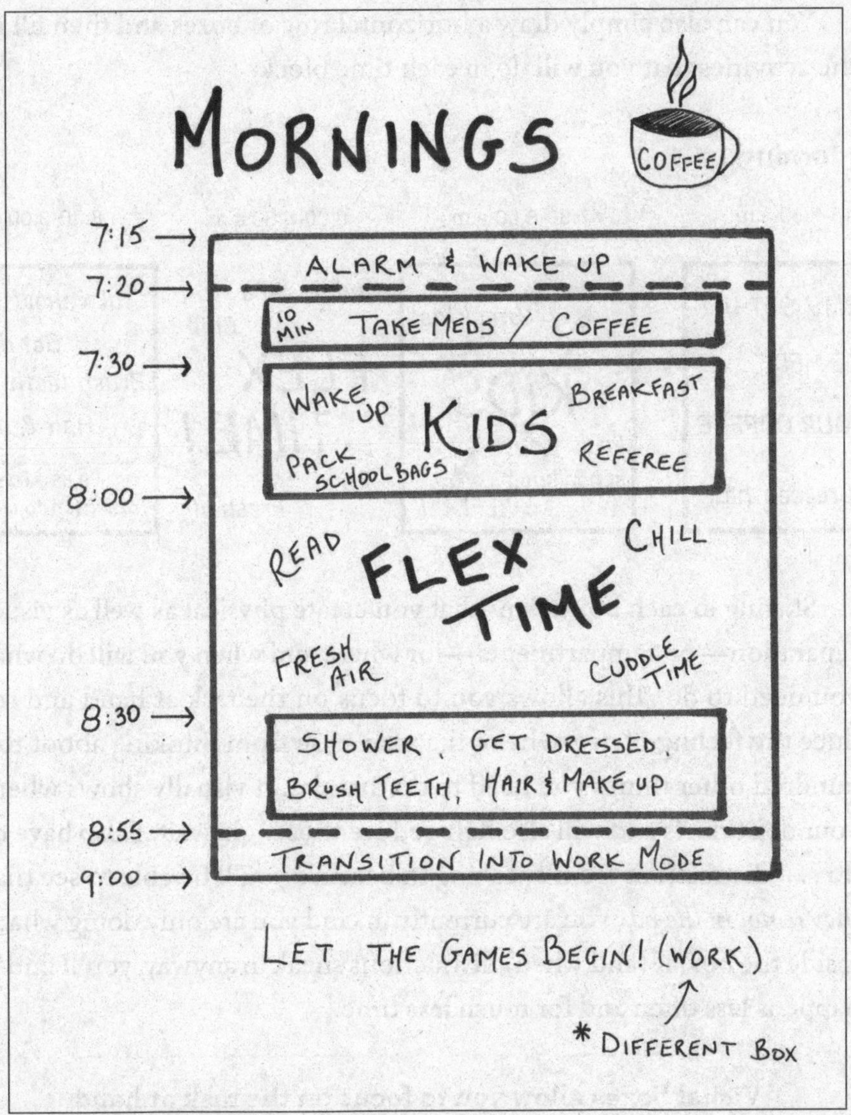

Eliza's Morning box was divided into all the things she needed to get done before work each day. Whether we have kids to take care of or not, we'll all have a different morning routine from Eliza's, but if you note the things you need to get done and designate them as activities in a box, plus factor in flex time (like the times you're already a bit more relaxed), you will have a plan ready. You'll also visually see how much time certain tasks take. I recommend you map out your boxes each night, so you have a visual to follow as soon as you wake up in the morning.

You can also simply draw a horizontal row of boxes and then fill in the activities that you will do in each time block.

Morning:

7:15-7:30 a.m.

ALARM / GET UP!
TAKE MEDS
POUR COFFEE
Breeeeathe...

7:30-8:00 a.m.

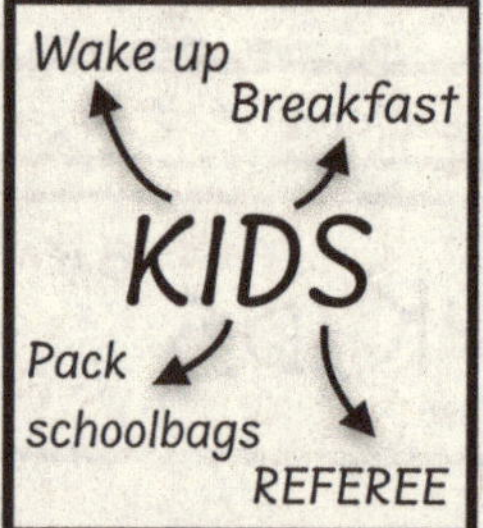

8:00-8:30 a.m.

Cuddle time
Chill
FLEX TIME!
Read
Fresh air

8:30-9:00 a.m.

Take shower
Get dressed
Brush teeth
Hair & makeup
8:55-9:00 a.m.
Transition to work mode

Staying in each box means that you create physical as well as visual separation—or compartments—for where and when you will do what you need to do. This allows you to focus on the task at hand and reduce the feeling of overwhelm that can arise from thinking about the hundred other things you need to do that day. It visually shows where your flex time is and will also help reduce those "oh, wait, I also have to do . . ." distractions from sneaking in because you'll be able to see that *they're not in the box* you are currently in, and you are only doing what's inside the box. If (and when) distractions sneak in anyway, you'll find it happens less often and for much less time.

> **Visual boxes allow you to focus on the task at hand and reduce the feeling of overwhelm that can arise from thinking about the hundred other things you need to do that day.**

Open (or Closed) for Business!

If you work from home, it's very easy to be interrupted by questions from your kids, requests from your partner, an invitation from a roommate, friends, household tasks, pets, your snack pantry, a TV screen, you name it. It's also extremely easy to feel that you're working *all the time* because there's no commute or specific office hours to denote when you are "at work." Or, if you make your own hours, just as there is no one to tell you when to work, there is no one to tell you when *not* to work! It's easy to stop working at noon, only to find yourself back on your laptop at 1:00 a.m. finishing the day's work when you should be sleeping. Every day can find you working for eighteen not-so-productive hours rather than seven or eight productive hours.

☑ To contain your workday, clarify your times by making a sign to put on your door or the back of your desk chair to clearly communicate to yourself (and others in your home) which hours you are busy "at work" and which hours you're not working (and available for others).

Ivy—Designing Office Hours

Ivy, an artist who works from home, has varying hours every day, which makes it challenging for her to separate work from her other responsibilities. She hung a small whiteboard on her door, where she posted her hours for the day and included different messages for her family at the bottom of the sign each day—"I love you all, but please do not *interrupt" or "Pretend I'm not really here and working at the gallery thirty minutes away!"*

Once everyone knows your schedule (including you), it is much easier to compartmentalize the times when you are working and when you are not. Also, if you are subject to the all-too-common ADHD ailment of "one-more-thing-itis"—that compulsive urge to finish "just one more thing" that ends up always taking longer than you thought—and it feels like you work 24–7 because you can never find your Stop button, it will help to put a clear end to your workday by creating a physical door sign for yourself, just like the signs you see in storefront windows that say: "Sorry, We Are Closed." Put this sign on the door to your home office, or put it on your computer screen or laptop, then physically walk away from your computer and get away from your work zone. Doing this will help you resist the temptation to do "just one more thing" for work, even if you have already stopped working for the day (*not that any of us do this*). The idea here is to create and communicate your designated times to do things. Having tangible visuals of those demarcations will help to compartmentalize what and when you do everything you need to do.

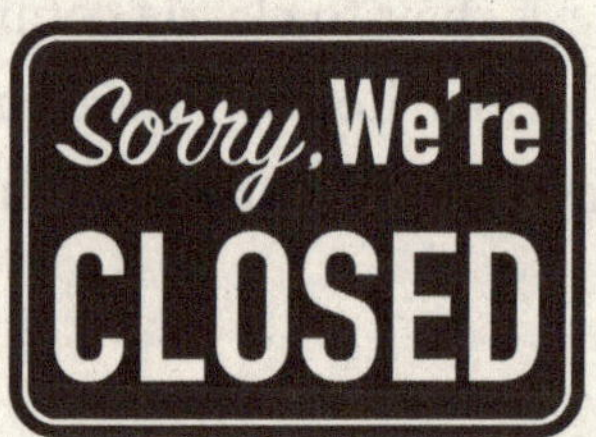

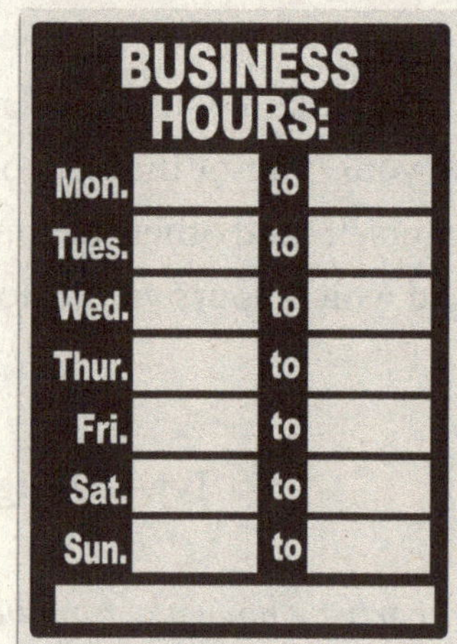

Separation of Space

Many of us are all too familiar with taking our laptops to the couch in the TV room, or the bedroom, or the kitchen table to work. In fact, it is so common, it feels completely normal. Unfortunately, this leads to us feeling like we're working 24–7 because every space in our lives is a work zone and all hours of the day are work times. With no separation between our work and personal space, along with having a brain that has difficulty creating separations, we're significantly increasing our nonstop experience of stress and overwhelm. There is no beginning or end.

If you always take your computer to bed with you to work on something, it's difficult to associate your bed with relaxation and sleep. The same with your family room. If your laptop is always there on the couch waiting for you to get back to what you were doing, it's much more difficult to be able to focus on your family.

☑ To start creating separation between work and personal spaces in your home, designate one area that's strictly off-limits for work—a room or spot where you commit to keeping your computer and any work-related items and activities out. This simple boundary can make a huge difference in helping you be fully present during downtime.

Nora—Constructing Walls

Nora is a building contractor who is self-employed. She literally builds walls for a living, but she did not have separation in any of the areas of her life. Because she didn't have an extra room to designate as an office, she was doing all her paperwork at the kitchen table so she could spread out, but was often distracted by her kids running through the kitchen to grab a snack, or noticing some aspect of housework that needed her attention.

In order to build some metaphorical walls, we looked at how to separate her day into Times (when) and Spaces (where), and what Category was going to fill each time and space (work, kids, health, friends, and so on). For Time, she marked out her work hours, housework hours, times for parenting responsibilities, and so on.

To create her separation in space, she set up a smaller table in the corner of her dining room for work. She even put a tiny plant and a small artistic wood carving that she loved on the table to designate it as an important space. When she sat down at that table, it was work, and only work, time. She successfully "built" walls to keep her responsibilities separated so she could give them the focus they needed.

Nora's "wall" kept her work and family life in separate zones in her home, which, to her surprise, led to having much more time to spend on each.

☑ Ritualize Your Transitions

Transition rituals are incredibly powerful and give your brain a concrete signal about making a physical and emotional shift from one thing to another.

You can create a set of actions or rituals that creates a transition cushion to help you move from one mode into another (like relaxation, work, friends, studying, or family mode). For example, when working from home, when it's time to transition to home/family mode, you could spend five minutes clearing your desk, shutting down your computer, or tucking in your chair and writing out what you will do the next day, or close the door and put out your "closed for business" sign. Or spend a few minutes listening to whatever music gets you into "home mode." If you're driving home, you could sit in your car in the driveway for two minutes and mentally go through the transition from work to home. You can set an intention for yourself for how you'd like your evening to be, you might choose a regular theme song to play as you transition from one life compartment to another—similar to the way your favorite show begins with its signature theme music and, when you hear it, you're instantly in the headspace of that show. Another way to mark an end to the workday is to change your clothes and wear something different for the evening portion of your day.

It doesn't matter what your action is; transition rituals are incredibly powerful and give your brain a concrete signal about making a physical and emotional shift from one thing to another—keeping the walls between them strong.

Once you develop the ability to create separations in your life and work, your experience of overwhelm will become much more manageable. Set separate zones and spaces for different activities, and do your best to do those activities *only* when in that zone or space: No work calls on date night. No texting with your friends while you're reading a story to your kids.

Knowing exactly what to do and when has never been easy for the ADHD brain, but reclaiming control of your time and space will ultimately give you more focus, clarity, and energy for all of it.

ADHD-Friendly Quick Summary

- Your incredible brain has a very hard time compartmentalizing, which leads to many of your ADHD symptoms—especially overwhelm.
- Without separation between thoughts, you are continually experiencing the ADHD reality of "everything all at once right now."

To start overcoming overwhelm:

- Simplify and narrow down action steps and concentrate on one area of focus at a time.
- Create easy-to-follow "recipes" for larger tasks by breaking them into a series of logical steps.
- Narrow down your to-do list to show only three items, then prioritize and single-handle each item without trying to multitask.

(continued on next page)

(continued from previous page)

To start creating separation in Time and Space:

- Build your own walls in your brain: Break your day into figurative time boxes.
- When working from home, create "Open for Business" and "Closed for Business" signs to communicate to yourself—and others—what hours you are (and are not) working.
- Create designated locations for separate activities.
- Establish a ritual that indicates the end of one mode or the beginning of another to clearly mark the transition in your brain.

ONE FOCUS

For those of us who struggle to create calm in our days, here's a simple, quick way to begin carving out that space—and time—for yourself:

Creating Separation at Home

Separate a Space: Create a separation in your personal space where you are *only* allowed to relax. No computer. No work. No housework. No communicating with people who aren't friends or family.

Pick a location of your choice: Is it an entire room in your home? Your bathtub? One specific couch? Is it a chair on a balcony? Is it in your car? Or a spot outdoors where you like to go (but maybe haven't been to in a while)? Choose what works best for you, but the key is to *never* bring anything but relaxation to your relaxation space. Herbal tea is allowed, work emails or your laptop are not.

Separate a Time: Now decide when the best time of day for you to do this will be. For one full week, spend five minutes per day in this spot as you "reinforce your walls" and practice bringing nothing but yourself and your intention to relax into this space. Give yourself a flexible time range in case you're in the middle of something when the scheduled time comes.

Set a daily reminder or an alarm on your phone to be sure you will take this important time for yourself. Example: Set a daily alarm for 9:00 p.m. reminding you that at some point in the next half hour you need to go to this space and relax for at least five minutes.

By maintaining this small separation you've created for yourself, you'll notice that after only one week, you will feel less overwhelmed by your "everything-all-at-once" internal reality, and you'll want to keep this time (or space) separated as much as possible.

17

Eliminate Disorganization and Chaos

Do you avoid inviting people to your home because of how messy it is? Are you always trying to find an empty space between different piles of stuff to stash more stuff? Do you use virtual or blurred backgrounds when videoconferencing because it would take too much time to make your real space presentable? Although many neurotypical people have the same struggles organizing their spaces, the difference is that there are specific ADHD factors that make organization a nonstop struggle for you, especially if you've been trying to address it the same way everyone else does.

For someone with ADHD, organization has to be approached from a different perspective and viewed as a means to an end: whether it's to create a calmer and less chaotic living space, to improve your efficiency and productivity, or simply to be on time for what's important because you'll no longer be held up looking for the various things you tend to misplace.

Every single ADHDer I've worked with struggles with organization in some area of their life. In fact, a lot of ADHDers are selectively disorganized! They may have a super-organized house or office but are constantly late for meetings or forget important dates, like birthdays and anniversaries. If you can keep things organized in some parts of your life, you're clearly not just a lazy slob who doesn't care. So what, then, is going on?

Following are some of the ways our most common ADHD symptoms can lead to challenges with organization.

- ***Impulsive behaviors*:** This is a big one. In the middle of doing one thing, you get inspired to tackle something else. Whatever you were doing is dropped wherever you are at that moment, and you skip to the next thing without another thought, leaving an unfinished mess behind.

- ***Procrastination or waiting until the last minute*:** Whether it's getting dressed for an event you're already late for or getting your materials together for a presentation, when you're always in a rush, totally behind, stressed out, and in catch-up mode, there's no time to think about where something "should" go or how you "should" be organizing your things or your space. The *only* thing that matters is getting *x*, *y*, and *z done*—and it's usually getting done at the very last minute, leaving total chaos in its wake.

- ***Being emotionally or mood-driven*:** Maybe the day comes when you get sick and tired of the disorder in your life and decide today is the day you will get everything organized. You watch three "get organized" videos online and read a full blog post written by today's most popular organization guru. With nothing more exciting to distract you, you jump right in! You make some progress, but the next day, you're over it. Why? Because the emotional frustration that motivated you to take action happened *yesterday*! Today, you're feeling totally fine about how things are, and you accept your mess as an integral part of your essence, so there's no push to change, especially when there are so many other more fun things you want to do instead.

- ***Being in constant overwhelm*:** You're motivated to straighten out your mess, but then when you think about everything you need to do to get it done, you freeze. You look at the space in question, and (once again!) you're like a deer caught in headlights. You have absolutely no idea where to begin. It's too much to handle right now. You're frozen, so you walk away to grab a snack or chat with your friend and forget all about it.

- ***Being noncommittal and indecisive*:** You're determined to get organized but can't stick with whatever systems you started to put in place, and it's equally difficult to make the decisions that come along with finding places to put things: *Do I put this here or over there? Why should it go over there when it also could be here?*

The same challenge goes for our classic just-in-case-er who thinks, *I need to hold on to this just in case someone else needs it.* The just-in-case-er is a wonderful and well-meaning person who keeps all options open and all their stuff available for everyone . . . never needing to decide or commit to what truly needs to go, just in case.

Aviva—The Just-in-Case Garage

Aviva, like many of us, has a million different interests, and she has accumulated a lot of stuff in her garage. There's old furniture she wants to refinish, yards of silk for learning Aerial Yoga, boxes of paint, paintbrushes, and canvases that she bought for art projects she meant to start years ago, loads of planting materials for her future backyard organic garden, and many boxes of who knows what that she saved for "just in case." Some of these items have been sitting in her garage for more than twenty years. For Aviva, the prospect of doing something with all her stuff raises too many questions and becomes completely overwhelming, so she holds on to everything. Just in case her kids eventually need the art supplies. Just in case her friend who just got a new place is looking for a chair exactly the size and style as the one in Aviva's garage. Just in case her schedule frees up and she suddenly finds the time to try Aerial Yoga. If she gets rid of the gardening supplies, will she never learn the art of organic gardening and be forced to eat pesticides in her food for the rest of her life? If she gets rid of any of these things, is she in fact throwing away the dreams she had for them and the possibilities they may have opened up for her life? Won't she be giving up on herself?

All these "just in case" thoughts keep Aviva in this never-ending limbo and her garage overflowing with more unused (but good!) stuff.

COUNTERINTUITIVE ORGANIZATION TIPS THAT WORK!

It's important for an ADHDer to view organization as a key step toward clearing out the external chaos in your life in order to create the time and space to get something more meaningful handled. It's like being able to find your car keys more easily so that you're not late for work—if you're going to build a path that takes you to having what you want and feeling how you want, you have to be able to access your path-building tools when you need them without spending your time and energy looking for them.

Our brains are wired to simultaneously resist and require organization! Regardless of the ways you're personally disorganized, you can learn to overcome it, clear your space (and your mind), and minimize the chaos in your life to get unstuck and move forward in the way that feels best for you!

Our brains are wired to simultaneously resist and require organization!

☑ Make Up Your Own Rules

Many people with ADHD have an underlying oppositional nature that makes it a challenge to follow other people's rules. Part of the problem with most organization systems is that they are full of "you must do this, and you have to do that," which, especially with organization, can trigger an emotional response reminiscent of when you were younger and heard things like, "*Why can't you just* put your socks away!" "Why do I have to keep telling you not to put your schoolbag there?" "You lost your homework (credit card, keys, phone) again?!" all while also telling you how to do it better—their way. It's enough to make anyone feel resistant. Plus, the recommendations you've been given by others are usually things that might work for neurotypical people but won't work for you.

If you tend to be oppositional by nature and you're an adult, you'll be much better off if you make up your own rules and do only what works for you! It's also usually much harder to break rules that you've created for yourself.

You can make rules for any organizational challenge. If your closet is overflowing to the point that you can't *ever* find what you're looking for, make some rules you know you'll follow. Maybe you can decide to donate one item of clothing for each new one you acquire. Or donate those items you know you've kept out of guilt—because you've never actually worn them. Or color-code and hang clothes next to similar-colored items to find them more easily the next time.

If important emails are always getting lost in the shuffle, establish rules for keeping them sorted so that nothing gets missed again. You can use email features like stars, flags, or color coding to visually categorize your emails into four priorities: 1.) immediately; 2.) later today; 3.) soon-ish; and 4.) whenever. Or limit when you check your emails and make a rule to only go through them at specific times each day so that your brain is turned "on" when it's time and you don't miss things, versus scrolling through your emails mindlessly in your pj's first thing in the morning before you have your first cup of coffee! The important thing is that *you* get to decide when and how you keep on top of them.

Here's another example: Let's say you are sick of wasting time *every single day* looking for what you need to get out the door in the morning. Here's how you could take the well-known organization strategy of designating a specific place or a "home" for things and customize it with your own rules. For example:

Your desired result: Not losing your keys or wallet, your phone, or your charger, or whatever it is you're *always* looking for at the last minute.

Create an easy and basic rule: Use a doorway basket ONLY for three or four specific essentials. Nothing else is allowed in the basket, ever.

Make it work for YOU: This is where you add the rules (or instructions) of your own. For example:

* Where will you put this basket so that you'll actually use it? On your entry table? Or, if you don't have a table, should you hang it on a hook near your door? Or, if you want to get stylish, search "entryway organizers," and you'll find lots of options. (If you're already on your way to looking these up, hopefully I'll see you again in a few hours.)
* What three or four essentials will you designate for that basket? Your essentials = can't leave home without them. Nothing else is allowed in that basket. Got it? *Nothing.* It's important that you're able to clearly see each of these items so they don't get lost under a pile of a hundred other things.
* Help yourself stick to your rule. If you can't stop yourself from dropping everything into the basket, then set a different rule that you'll check the basket each night to remove all nonessential items. Or you can put a sticky note on or next to the basket with a list of the items that are supposed to go in there. As soon as you come home and are at your door, the

> visual you've created tells you exactly what to do. No decisions need to be made; there's no searching around wondering where to put whatever you have with you. It's one less thing for your overcrowded brain to deal with. *Ahhh, serenity.*

This is just one example of a system. After using *any* system that you customize for yourself consistently for a few days, you'll have it down.

☑ Make It as Entertaining as Possible

Make organizing somewhat enjoyable so you'll be motivated to continue! Beyond simply listening to your favorite music, incorporate whatever's fun or entertaining whenever you're organizing. Some of our client favorites are:

- Organize your space while wearing your running shoes and workout clothes. Doing this seems to automatically put people into a "Just Do It!" mindset.
- Make a video of yourself talking about the random stuff that you find while you're cleaning up.
- Arrange to talk to a friend at the time you both decide to organize.
- Assign points to tackling areas (1 drawer = 5 points) where a certain number of points = doing something else you want to do (20 points = take a break, eat a Popsicle, play your guitar, check your texts, whatever you consider to be a reward).
- Grab a pair of dice that you can roll to tell yourself what task to do (e.g., roll a 1 = organize the top desk drawer, roll a 5 = make the bed, roll a 6 = do the dishes, etc.).

Truly anything goes. Whatever makes it more interesting for you, as long as you *do* one of them rather than just reading about it.

☑ Use Time Blasts

Dividing organization tasks into tiny sprints is one of the simplest ways to overcome internal and external chaos. Instead of thinking, *I have to spend Sunday afternoon organizing my home office*, flip your time frame and say, "How much of my desk can I organize in the next two minutes?" (We affectionately call this the Two-Minute Tidy.) Or if that feels too long, try forty-five seconds. Then set a timer and ready, set, go! You will be surprised at how much you can get done.

This Time Blast approach works not only for organizing spaces but also for organizing your calendar, your phone contacts, your emails, or the files on your computer. Give yourself a small amount of time and go for it. Play around with Newton's first law of motion! For the ADHD brain, getting started is often the hardest part. But once you get started, your brain will connect with the energy of the momentum, and your actions will almost always automatically follow.

☑ Break It into Tiny Spaces

I know how difficult it can be to get started on almost anything, especially when it's big or you don't know where or how to start. It never fails: the second you begin thinking about organizing one thing, your mind is immediately flooded with twenty other areas that also need your attention, and they all need it now. The enormity of the task is now so overwhelming that you give up on doing anything at all. So, unless you're someone who works best in large blocks of time, do not, by any means, think about organizing your *entire* living room, office, or garage in one day. Even if it seems like a *reeeally* great idea at the time. Instead, think about just one shelf, one surface, one corner of one shelf, or one small section of the floor. Once you have picked it out in your mind, cut it in half. Now cut it in half again. And again. At this point, you're staring at what seems like a ridiculously small space to organize—so small that it might seem completely pointless.

Why bother? What difference will it make? Let me tell you, it will make all the difference. The difference it makes *isn't* in the space in the room. IT'S. IN. YOUR. BRAIN.

☑ Keep Your Brain Winning!

For the ADHD brain that tends to be mood-driven, taking advantage of the feeling you get from WINNING works wonders. Remember, tasks will always get done when you break them down into minuscule pieces so small that you *100 percent* can succeed at them without fail. No matter how small, that feeling of success and accomplishment leads to the emotional motivation you need to tackle the rest of the space—one tiny bit at a time.

After you've selected a small section to organize, and taken care of it, you can move on to the next tiny section. Then you can do that same process over and over again and be successful every single time! You'll find that you can accomplish a lot—usually much more than you would if you tried to think about tackling the entire thing at once.

The Bite-Size Mini Habit: A similar approach is to get in the habit of taking a repeatable action toward getting organized, even if it seems really, really small. For example, each time you walk into your office, clear one or two items. Every time you leave your car, take out one or two items, and so on. It's small, and it may feel insignificant; yet it's all in the name of winning.

☑ One Thing Now Is Better Than Everything Never

You know from experience, and from previous chapters, that if you try to do twenty things all at the same time, none of them will get done. However, if you focus your energy on attacking one little corner right now, you *will* get to those other spaces.

Approach any space you want to organize as if you are looking through a cardboard paper towel tube. Whatever you see through that small aperture is what you will tackle now: the top-right corner of your desk, one part of one drawer in your bathroom, one shelf in your kitchen, or one thing you need to put away that you've been walking past all week and not putting away, and so on. Next week, you'll tackle another space, like your closet, one small section at a time. Eventually, everything will come together if you just focus on one small and simple area at a time. I promise.

Approach any space you want to organize as if you are looking through a cardboard paper towel tube. Whatever you see through that small aperture is what you will tackle now.

I know that your ADHD brain might be already pushing back against these approaches, and you might be telling yourself that they're too obvious and simple. First, know that for ADHD, simple is good! These ideas are tried and tested. Remember, you don't have to commit to any approach for forever. Just commit to one for one week, or even two days if that's easier to swallow. Try it out for real, and if it doesn't make your life better, scrap it and go back to the way things were before.

But let's say it does work and your life gets easier. Try applying the same method to something else. Creating your own rules, keeping it entertaining, and following tiny-step approaches that work for organization and your ADHD brain will help you to minimize overwhelm and stress while also increasing the overall feeling of calm and control that you have in your life.

ADHD-Friendly Quick Summary

- Being organized is an important step toward accomplishing something more meaningful, like eliminating the stress, chaos, and frustration in our lives.

(continued on next page)

(continued from previous page)

- Many of your most prevalent ADHD symptoms are what lead to your organizational challenges.
- For those of us with a more oppositional nature, creating your own rules for organization and customizing them is the best way to have rules in your life that you'll want to follow.
- Make organizing as entertaining as you can.
- When starting to get organized, pick the smallest place to begin so that it takes up less space in your brain.
- Keep Your Brain WINNING! Once you have successfully completed one small space, continue organizing one more tiny space at a time, then another and another.

ONE FOCUS

Stick to One, and Get It Done

Choose anything that you'd like to be better organized—your kitchen counter, a bathroom drawer, your inbox, the surface of your desk—whatever causes you the most distress when you look at it.

Take a "before" picture of the space, and then zoom in to choose a tiny area within that space to work on for now.

Set a timer for a two-minute Time Blast and go! Declutter as much of that tiny space as you can within the time limit. After the Time Blast, write down in your notebook approximately how many square feet or inches, or number of messages in your inbox, you were able to tackle. Do this every day for five days in a row. After day five, take an "after" picture to remind you of what you have accomplished in less than a week! If you have a home printer, print the after picture (on regular paper is fine) to tape in your notebook or your Wall of Attention as a visual reminder.

18

Manage Your Time to Manage Your Life

How you spend your time is how you spend your life. Your lifetime is a collection of minutes and hours, and how you spend them ends up being what comprises your life. Many of us typically spend hours every day on things that might feel good in the short term but don't move us forward and ultimately take us away from what we want. We can spend hours on social media, watching TV, debating with people, daydreaming, and scrolling on our phones, tablets, or laptops "researching," playing games, or watching random videos about things that won't ever mean anything to us.

How you spend your time is how you spend your life.

Most ADHDers have a difficult relationship with time. Time blindness, in addition to the ability to hyper-focus when you're deeply engaged in something, can cause you to think you've only spent an hour on something without realizing that it's literally been most of the day, so you forgot to eat lunch, missed dinner, and were supposed to be somewhere else ages ago. Or it can allow time to stretch endlessly while waiting for something where you feel like you can't control your impatience any longer, but when you check your watch, it has—impossibly—been only thirty-one seconds.

Our internal clocks seem to fluctuate from moving super fast to being in stall mode or not working at all. We often don't realize what time it is and are completely unable to estimate how long something will (or did) take. We also tend to get lost in daydreaming, or hyper-focusing on something so intently that time doesn't seem to exist. And some of us even come to believe that time isn't important because we are *always* late, and it's just expected of us.

Believe it or not, although it may feel as if you are being controlled by some powerful external force playing with the passage of time and pulling you into inescapable rabbit holes, you can learn to be conscious of time and to do things in a way that helps you use the limited time you have on the things that matter most to you. In addition to what we talked about in chapter 16, here are some tried and tested techniques to help you prioritize and leverage time to your advantage.

TAKE BACK YOUR TIME

It's a symptom of our culture and society that we all feel we're running out of time, but for those with ADHD, this feeling is much more acute. When you are trying to get things done and it seems that there aren't enough hours in the day, plus everything feels like it has the exact same weight of importance and you don't know what to do first, it's helpful to take a step back and get clear on your priorities.

☑ Two Hours a Day

Imagine that you were told by your doctor that you could only work for a maximum of two hours per day and not one second more. Without overthinking it, what you'd choose to do in those two hours each day to reach your goals as quickly as possible are likely your highest-value tasks. You'll also likely discover that overanalyzing, over-researching, perfecting, impulsively jumping from task to task, and spending time on your social media feeds won't make the list.

Take a few minutes to respond to the following prompts in your notebook:

- What are the two or three tasks that you would choose to do if you only had two hours a day to get stuff done?
- Break one of the tasks down into very small and guaranteed-doable steps.
- Put the tiny doable steps into your calendar so you know you'll actually do them and move forward on each step until your high-value task is accomplished. You can then do the same for the other tasks you chose.

What are the two or three tasks that you would choose to do if you only had two hours a day to get stuff done?

Knowing what is of value is essential, but you still need to figure out how to best manage your time so that you can act on those high-value tasks.

☑ Time Categories

Write down how and where you mostly spend your time (and your life): work, food and meal prep, sleep, time with kids, exercise, reading, time with your partner, volunteering, going out with friends, chatting with friends online, paying bills, family outings, gaming, housekeeping, excessive shopping, social media, TV, managing expenses, hobbies, and so on.

Next, in your notebook, sort all these activities into the following three categories:

***Must Do*:** Work, eat, sleep, be with your kids, pay your bills, exercise, spend time with your partner, family time, and so on.

***Should or Like to Do*:** Socializing, hobbies, outings, volunteering, and so on.

Time Wasters: (All the things you get sucked into for longer than you want.) Social media, gaming, excessive shopping, watching TV, and so on.

You can probably predict that many of us end up spending a lot of our time (and life) in the Time Wasters category, simply because those activities don't require much thought or energy, and they're the easiest to fall into.

☑ Where *Does* the Time Go?

If you don't already know where you commonly spend your time, find out. For just the next two days, track your time as billable hours the way a lawyer or a consultant does. Every hour or so, note what you did in the previous sixty minutes. Color-code or label whether each activity was a Must Do, a Should or Like to Do, or a Time Waster.

The tasks you wrote down don't represent every activity you do, but writing them out will give you an idea of what to keep as your top priorities. Also, many of us confuse the Must Do category with Like to Do. For example, "I am going to stop working on this manuscript because I *have* to drive to that specialty food shop to get the really *good* pasta to cook tonight." Yes, dinner has to happen, but maybe it can be something simple (or takeout). Always keep in mind that the Must Do category represents your nonnegotiables, or things you'd do if you only had "two hours a day" to do anything.

☑ Time Tools

Now, choose one of your Must Do tasks. Let's say it's exercising. You then need to make sure that you can set aside the time to guarantee that you're able to exercise. This is obviously easier said than done, which is why you need to have tools.

There are a number of tools to help you manage your tasks and activities, including calendars, timers, reminders, and alarms, but you have to make sure to use them in an ADHD-friendly way, which will be different for all of us.

- **Calendar** (computer, paper, planner, whiteboard, phone)—choose the one that will be *easiest* for you to use.
    - Treat your calendar as a "sacred" place for important commitments.
    - Make sure all your digital calendars are synced (work and personal, computer and phone).

- **Digital reminder or alarm** (buzzing, ringing, music)—whichever one you won't ignore.

- **A "high impact" Message** in your reminders and alarms that you'll pay attention to.

- **Timer** (visual countdown timer, phone).

- **Your Parking Lot** notepad for setting aside distractions (explained below).

☑ Your Sacred Calendar (and How to Use It)

In ancient civilizations, calendars were literally carved in stone and meticulously created over long periods of time in order to track agricultural cycles and religious events: basically, what we believed to be entirely responsible for life and death. Now, if only we took our calendars this seriously—we'd never miss a thing!

Your calendar is one of the most useful tools you have, but only if you treat it as *sacred*. Meaning that if something is in your calendar, you need to make it happen. To keep your reasons for setting aside this time front and center, you'll need to *add emotional weight* to entries with a note to remind you of *why* you are doing this activity. For example: The word *Exercise* in your calendar on Tuesday morning between 7:00 and 8:00

a.m. can easily be, and often is, totally ignored. Try including emotional detail. For example, on my client Sari's calendar, on Monday, Wednesday, and Friday at 7:00 a.m., it says, "*Exercise! Or keep feeling like crap and be angry at my body and my lazy-butt self for the rest of my life!*" It's harsh, but she's a lighthearted, funny woman who honestly has a healthy relationship with her body, and the harsh messages are in her own words and work for her. For you, write whatever message gives *you* a strong kick in the butt, in *your* own words. You can also use emotionally charged messages when you set reminders and alarms on your phone.

☑ Structured Work Sessions

To stay productive and focused while working on something, you can set up your working time in a structured manner, a.k.a. Structured Work Sessions (SWS). This is a modified and more flexible ADHD-friendly version of the Pomodoro Technique, which involves sandwiching our breaks with timed work sessions.

Basically, you are going to structure specific focused working sessions around active *timed* breaks (this is important!). You will also be creating a metaphorical Parking Lot to keep any distractions at bay (also important!).

Structure specific focused working sessions around active *timed* breaks.

To put your Structured Work Session into action, you'll need a timer and a separate notebook (or a few blank pages at the end of the notebook that you've already been using) to serve as your Parking Lot.

- First, choose an amount of time for your focused work periods as well as for your break periods. For example, you may decide to have two forty-five-minute work sessions interrupted by a ten-minute physical action break (45/10/45). Adjust your time frame to what works for your brain: if longer stretches of time are more effective, you could do 90/20/90, or if shorter bursts work better, you can try 15/3/15. Whatever is best for you!

- Select which activities you will engage in during your breaks. Playing music, stair climbing, push-ups, playing with your dog, going outside, or taking a short walk are all viable options.
- Use your timer for your work time *and* your break time. It's important to have a hard stop for your breaks so they don't last all day. For your ten- (or twenty-, or three-) minute activity break, it's best to physically move your body—this will legitimately "refresh" your brain! Don't just stay sitting in front of your computer or phone on social media or some other online distraction.
- Park your distractions: Keep a "Parking Lot" notebook and a pen right next to you to manage distracting thoughts that would otherwise interrupt your workflow.

☑ Your Parking Lot (and How to Use It)

The Parking Lot is a notebook that you keep beside you so you can write down, or "park," the "interruption thoughts" that distract you while you are working on something else. It's a necessary tool to help keep you focused on the task at hand when you have a sudden thought (or thirty), new ideas, or inspirations that threaten to take you off course and down a rabbit hole of unproductivity, potentially sidetracking you for hours! Recording your interruption thoughts in a designated space that you can access later gives these important yet ill-timed thoughts and ideas the love and respect they deserve. Your brain will feel that the thought has been acknowledged without having to spend two hours unabashedly devoted to it, and you will be able to maintain continued focus on what you're doing!

Recording your interruption thoughts in a designated space that you can access later gives these important yet ill-timed thoughts and ideas the love and respect they deserve.

☑ You've Been on Time Before, Really!

Being late is a great example of a repeat offender with time management because it tends to happen *a lot* for many of us. We're not only late for work but for events we're legitimately excited about—like a dinner date, our kid's performance, or meeting up with friends.

Besides time blindness and our tendency to get lost in hyper-focus, another common reason for us often being late is our struggle with "one-more-thing-itis"—that compulsion we mentioned in chapter 16, where there's always just one more thing we absolutely have to do that seems to put us on the wrong side of being on time.

Regardless of why you tend to be late, you can connect with the part of you that's able to be on time. Think about occasions when you *were* on time—they have probably happened more often than you think. Maybe for flights, weddings, interviews, exams, medical appointments?

1. Where were you going?
2. What were you doing?
3. Why was it important to be on time?
4. What did you actually, factually, *do* to be on time?
5. What did you *not* do so that you would be on time?

Maybe you listened to your alarm when it went off the first time? Maybe you resisted the urge to do that one last thing? Or maybe you set something up the night before, like choosing your outfit ahead of time so it'd be easier to get ready for that event.

When you remember how you have managed to be on time in the past, you will realize that if you have done it before (yes, you have—fact!), even if it was challenging, you can do it again.

SETTING BOUNDARIES FOR YOURSELF

Many of us feel like we're always living in reaction mode, totally at the whim of other people and external circumstances. Sometimes we're not able to manage our time, or be on time, because we're so busy doing things for everyone else, making it nearly impossible to have the time for what *we* need. Setting boundaries will help you to clarify what you want, and don't want, to spend your time doing.

Maybe you're a people pleaser or a bit of a chameleon who finds it hard to be true to herself. Your heart is absolutely in the right place, but you can be pulled in multiple directions at once, leaving you without the time or space to think about what you need to be doing—or where you need to be!

But let's say you have goals for yourself and you'd like to be able to start spending time on them. You can start by first setting some *internal boundaries*. This means sticking to what YOU most want to do and not being swayed by the influence of those around you.

☑ Saying Yes or No?

Saying "yes" to something = saying "no" to something else, just like saying "no" to something = saying "yes" to something else. For example, saying "yes" to staying late at work = saying "no" to having dinner with your spouse. Saying "no" to another late-night TV episode = saying "yes" to getting more sleep. You get to choose what to say "yes" to, which will help you say "no" or "not yet" to other things that might suck up your time and energy. Doing this frees you up to focus on your own goals so that you can say "yes" to yourself and what you've been wanting to accomplish.

Saying "yes" to something = saying "no" to something else, just like saying "no" to something = saying "yes" to something else.

If you're a perpetual people pleaser, and you know it's eating up your (life)time, practice saying "no" (or something equivalent) once or twice a day when people ask you to do things. For example: "I would like to give this some thought before I commit." Or, "Let me get back to you by tomorrow." Or, "I don't think I can do that right now."

Veronica—Where Is the Fire?

Veronica is a very busy, very scattered executive at a job that seemed to constantly put her in crisis mode and needing to put out fires—hers and everyone else's. Nearly anytime someone raised an issue, she shifted her attention to that current fire, but then another crisis would arise, and she was pulled into dealing with that one. She was helping others, but this wasn't allowing her to work on her own prioritized tasks.

Although she needed to be responsive to clients' and coworkers' needs, her personal participation wasn't always essential when someone raised an alarm. To get a better sense of what truly needed her time and attention, we asked Veronica to start keeping note of what was genuinely an urgent issue that only she could respond to, versus a perceived fire that didn't necessarily require her personal time. This real versus perceived distinction is huge*—especially because we perceive most "fires" as catastrophic.*

Additionally, to help her stay on track, we had Veronica write down her top priority for the day in bold letters and put it where she could easily see it. If she got pulled off task, she had a visual reminder of what she needed to return to once she was done putting out someone else's fire. At the end of each workday, she took an objective inventory of the daily fires and assessed if they were real or perceived. This new information helped her to separate and clarify what she needed to take care of, from what other people were pulling her into.

Keeping her priority list front and center, combined with her analysis of real versus perceived emergencies, allowed Veronica to set simple boundaries and say "no" (in a nice way) without guilt when someone approached her with a fire that wasn't a real emergency that only she could handle. More importantly, she discovered that once her colleagues learned to respect her boundaries, they quickly started handling most of their "emergencies" without her.

Managing time is often challenging for those with ADHD—whether you are chronically late, get lost in what you are doing (thank you, hyper-focus), or have no idea how long things take. When you implement the tools and actions to help you become aware of how you spend your time and how to better manage it, you'll be on your way to controlling how you choose to spend your minutes and days—and ultimately how you choose to spend your life!

ADHD-Friendly Quick Summary

- How you spend your time is how you spend your life.
- ADHDers tend to struggle with time management because of challenges with how we estimate time, our tendency to get lost in hyper-focus, and our compulsive need to finish "just one more thing."
- The tasks you would do if you only had two hours a day are likely your top priority or highest-value tasks.
- Become conscious of your specific time waster activities.

(continued on next page)

(continued from previous page)

- Use tools like calendars, timers, and reminders to not only plan how and when to use your time but to be sure that you remember to follow through on what you want to do.
- Treat your calendar as sacred. If it's in your calendar, you must do it.
- Design your own Structured Work Sessions in time periods that work for you.
- Remember to time your breaks (*and do something physical!)* and use your Parking Lot for distraction management.
- Set strong internal boundaries so that you can make decisions quickly about saying "yes" or "no" to demands on your time.

ONE FOCUS

Completing Your Highest-Value Tasks

First thing each morning, make a super-short to-do list with just two or three high-priority items on it. These can be the items you would choose to do if you only had two hours a day to do anything.

Break these items down into tiny mini-steps, and *single handle each one until complete*. You can use time management tools like Structured Work Sessions, timers, reminders, alarms, and a Parking Lot to keep you on track. As you complete each step, check it off the list and feel free to put a smiley face beside the completed item.

At the end of the day, post your completed steps where you'll see them—this is great if you ever *feel* like you didn't end up getting anything done.

Do this for five days, and then review how much you did!

19

Conquer Procrastination and Get It Done

Frankly, the subject of procrastination could take up this entire book. Everyone, and I mean everyone, procrastinates. We all have tasks that we'd rather not deal with—taxes, cleaning up after our pets, scheduling car maintenance, doing laundry, taxes (still!), and on and on. Procrastination is not unique to people with ADHD but how—and how often—it impacts us *is*, so the way your incredible brain needs to address and overcome procrastination is unique as well.

THE PROCRASTINATION MYTH

Procrastination is one of the stereotypes most often associated with ADHD, yet the root causes of this behavior are, unfortunately, largely misunderstood. There's a popular belief that people with ADHD procrastinate because they're waiting for that "last-minute" adrenaline rush to get something done under pressure, which aligns with the stereotype of ADHDers being hyperactive adrenaline junkies; and although this is true for some, it's not at all true for most of us.

In my experience working exclusively with adults with ADHD, the reason the majority of us procrastinate is *not* our love of last-minute stimulus to get us into gear but because of our faithful partner in crime *overwhelm*, which causes us to not know where or how to start on a task in the first place! This leads to you putting off projects and spending most of your time on anything *else* that's easier just to escape (or ignore) your overwhelm! The more time that passes, the more the thing you are putting off feels out of reach and undoable.

The reason the majority of us procrastinate is *not* our love of last-minute stimulus to get us into gear but because of our faithful partner in crime *overwhelm*, which causes us to not know where or how to start on a task in the first place!

This is exactly how procrastination can derail you for weeks, months, or even years at a time. You start with every intention of accomplishing something, and yet when it's time to take action, your brain freezes, and you do, too. To break the paralysis, your brain unconsciously seeks out something easier and more interesting! Maybe it's chatting with a close friend? Finally trying out that recipe you got from someone last year—it sounded doable and you need to make dinner anyway. Designing a home page for your new website? Finally putting your winter clothes in storage now that it's July? Maybe it's researching clever life hacks—*Oh, look . . . I can de-wrinkle my clothes with ice cubes when I accidentally leave them in the dryer overnight!* These things serve as Band-Aids for the feeling of overwhelm, but they do nothing to solve it. The tasks you've been putting off will still be there tomorrow. And because more time has passed, they'll often feel bigger and more overwhelming than before.

Eventually, usually the night before something important is due or scheduled to happen, your brain's ride-or-die pal, good old stimulus, shows up at your door. That stimulus, fueled by panic and urgency, is so strong that it overrides the overwhelm that was keeping you stuck and, as stimulus usually does, gives you the focus to get whatever you need done. Because you weren't "hoping for" or enjoying the stimulus that shows up, it's super stressful! And once you finish doing whatever it was that you were putting off, by the next day, you feel more stressed out, overwhelmed, and depleted than you did initially, which makes it that much harder to start the next thing.

THE EFFECTS OF OVERWHELM AND FEAR

A few prevalent factors contribute to your procrastination tendencies. Do any of the following resonate with you?

Big Emotion

This is the most common reason ADHDers procrastinate on big projects. When something is important, it becomes a gigantic deal in your mind, taking on more and more emotional significance until it feels unmanageable. With so much at stake, the project gets pushed off or maybe never even gets started.

Anoushka—Delaying Her Dissertation

Anoushka had been working on her dissertation for more than two years, diligently devoting time to it every day. However, most of that time has been spent thinking, worrying, and stressing about it, and she had very little written. Anoushka is highly intelligent and had identified a variety of directions she could take for the paper, but anytime she got close to choosing one, she would second-guess herself, wondering if another option was better and contemplating all the different ways she could restructure the entire thing. She was constantly consumed by this project, but because she wasn't getting words down on the page, she was freaking out that she wasn't making any progress.

The hours she spent in front of the computer (although she was often scrolling through social media) and the constant circular thoughts she has about the paper make her feel like she's working on it nonstop. But once I began having her measure how many hours she spent overanalyzing and rethinking the theme of her paper, compared to how many hours she actually spent writing, she realized she had to do things differently. To get out of her head, while already knowing the massive effort she had already put into planning the outline of her paper, we had her start focusing on writing just one sentence at a time within a certain amount of time. Her limit was two minutes per sentence. One sentence led to another, and she quickly started making progress and building her momentum, until she was finally able to reach the finish line.

Fear and Procrastination

You'd almost never guess by looking at someone seemingly in a great mood doing something enjoyable like binge-watching a TV show, relaxing to their favorite music, making a complicated yet delicious meal, or indulging in a spontaneous shopping spree, but for many of us, there are pervasive fears running in the back of our minds that cause us to delay our most meaningful tasks indefinitely while we take refuge in our favorite and more comfortable distractions.

Fear of Failure or Looking Bad

There's always the possibility of not doing something well enough, being wrong, or letting others down. As discussed in part 2, this fear of failing can be debilitating. Rather than declare your project Done! and subject it to scrutiny that could find it lacking, you push the finish line further and further away by spending excessive amounts of time on research and working in perfection mode. And perfectionism, because it looks like thoughtful, responsible behavior, is one of the most intelligent ways for people to procrastinate, yet can easily result in never finishing (or even starting) what you need to do.

Fear of Success

This fear can be stronger than the fear of failure and is an equally common reason for us to procrastinate. Just the thought of the expectations that others might have of you, and the new responsibilities that will come with success, is unbearably overwhelming. What happens if you do an amazing job at what you're taking on? What if you're asked to do it again? "Wouldn't I have *more* work to do? Won't I eventually disappoint them?" Putting off what you're working on protects you from setting a standard that you may not be able to live up to and the pressure that goes along with it!

Fear of Breaking Your Stride

You know you need to start that important thing, but you have other *less* urgent things to do and worry about getting them done, too. Based on how well you know yourself, you're worried that if you stop the smaller tasks to start on the more important task, you'll never be able to get back to what you were originally doing! The overwhelming fear of stopping, or that you'll forget to finish what you're currently doing, takes over. Instead of pausing to work on the bigger things, you stick with whatever you were already doing, and the truly critical tasks go to the back of the line.

You may have experienced one or more of these factors that cause overwhelm, fear, and consequent procrastination. That said, knowing what you're up against can make a huge difference in helping you to move forward.

HOW TO NOT PUT THINGS OFF UNTIL TOMORROW, AND THE NEXT DAY, AND THE DAY AFTER THAT

To overcome procrastination, you need to cut through the overwhelm of the task—and the emotions surrounding it—to make it easier to start in the first place, and then implement the strategies that help you to be in action and get it done. Here's how.

VERB-ALIZE IT

Anyone can enter events into a calendar, but for adults with ADHD who want an extra push to get things done, we need to tell ourselves exactly what to do, using verbs! Our brains can easily ignore and postpone generic ideas, but clear spoken or written action words in our calendar will instantly create direction and emotional movement.

☑ When you're feeling overwhelmed by anything you need to do, enter it in your calendar as an action and make it *specific*. For example, instead of entering "Midterm exam prep," add "*Write out* four exam flash cards before study group." Instead of "Sales meeting presentation," write "*Develop* one marketing strategy with my sales team." Instead of "Workout," write "*Go to* (name of) yoga class at (name of) studio." Basically, every task in your calendar should be preceded by a verb. A written action or direction that pushes you into motion without giving your mind any space to think around it.

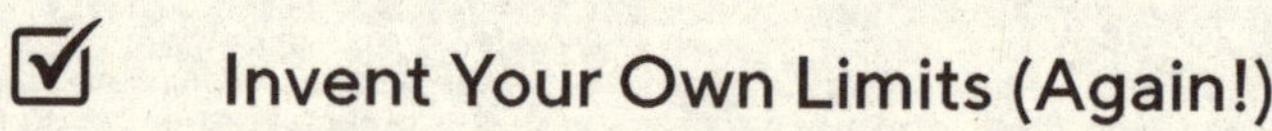

Every task in your calendar should be preceded by a verb.

☑ Invent Your Own Limits (Again!)

ADHDers are excellent at jumping into what's urgent because urgency is a stimulus that overrides overwhelm. However, when something isn't urgent (even if it's important) or if it doesn't have much meaning for you, then anything and everything else can take precedence. If the big goal is an open-ended task with no due date, it's much less likely to get done. You can overcome this by creating simple limits for yourself, and when it's your personal system, there is a much better chance of it working for you. That said, you have to keep it realistic and make sure the limit is doable. Imagine you are *only* allowed ten minutes to work on this project—how much can you get done? Or put a quantity limit on what you are doing—decide to write or read *only* three pages, or *only* brainstorm a maximum of five options for summer vacation or three possible restaurants to take your friend on their birthday, and so on. The magic words here are *only five* or *only three*. The specific limits and rules are yours to create and will help you focus on getting something done without letting it expand into something unmanageable.

☑ Create a Perfectionism Limit

As noted earlier, I really believe that perfectionism is one of the "smartest" ways for humans to procrastinate. I mean, who can fault a brilliant mind striving for true excellence? If perfectionism often stalls you, you may be someone who's very intelligent and, as mentioned with our overthinkers in chapter 10, in some ways, even "too smart for your own good."

Your procrastination doesn't usually take the form of flaking off, lying around in your sweats sipping mai tais. (Not that there's anything wrong with that.) Your preferred modes of procrastination might be quite astute and involve over-researching and taking fascinating deep dives into the project you're working on, where you go so far from your original focus that you might actually lose track of what you're supposed to be working on—sometimes before you even start.

Just as you can create your own time constraints, you can also set your own research limitations. For example: Set a timer for a maximum of forty minutes for research, and when time is up, you have to *start* on the first paragraph, or make one reservation for your vacation, or make that purchase . . . regardless of how unprepared you may feel.

Beyond being unable to start on things, your perfectionism also can delay you from *finishing* something. Whatever you're doing has to be perfect before you can finish it, and you can honestly keep perfecting it forever, while it never ends up getting done—which defeats the entire purpose of doing it in the first place. So you also need to set a limit to finish, since perfectionists almost never feel that anything is quite complete.

☑ Make It 90 Percent Good Enough!

If you feel that nothing is ever good enough to be "done," challenge yourself to play with the idea of doing things imperfectly (at "only" a 90 percent level) for just a day or two. Think of it as living in "first draft" mode. Try it in at least one area of your life—even at work! (Well, maybe not at work if you're a brain surgeon.) As most of us are not neurosurgeons, it won't take long to realize that nothing is going to fall apart if you turn in a project or do a task at a 90 percent level. (After all, 90 percent is still an A, right?) Loosening your grip on perfection and letting things go even if you know you could potentially make them even better (whether or not it *needs* to be better) will free you up to move forward and finally get your stuff done.

☑ Remember Your Big Why

Because we're emotionally driven, women with ADHD are less likely to procrastinate on meaningful things. If what you're procrastinating on doesn't have a lot of emotion (even if it's important), or energy, or purpose behind it, you'll be distracted by anything else that draws your attention, and it will be easy for the project to get completely lost in the crowd.

Sometimes it only takes a few minutes to reconnect yourself to the Big Why behind what you've been procrastinating on. You can attach even your smallest projects to a bigger purpose by writing in your notebook: "I need to start (insert task), *so that I can* __________ (your Big Why)."

INTERRUPT YOUR DISTRACTIONS

As we saw with Anoushka, it's possible that you often feel you're working on something tirelessly, when in fact, you're procrastinating! Maybe you're on your computer but getting lost in the endless abyss of the internet, or you're working alongside other people and getting distracted by continuous social interactions, or perhaps you're frequently taking two-hour-long extended breaks to "quickly" check your phone for a minute or grab a snack from the kitchen. If part of your mind is on what you're trying to do but your actions are in a totally different place, it'll help to put systems in place to get you refocused so that another month doesn't slip by without your task getting done.

☑ Here are some effective interruptions to help you move forward on what you need to be doing:

1. Write yourself a message that says: "Am I working on (task X) right now?" Put the note somewhere visible (like right on the corner of your computer screen, on your fridge, your TV remote, or your phone screen) so you will see it often to remind you to stay on task.
2. Set an alarm on your phone to go off every ninety minutes with a personal reminder message like "Make sure I'm doing ______!"
3. If you check email regularly, schedule and send emails to yourself for specific times of day to remind you of what you're supposed to be doing at this time so the push to stay on track is staring at you from your inbox.

Use whatever method and words speak to you. These purposeful interruptions can be super helpful at distracting you from your distractions.

With the help of the tools above, you can focus on being able to simply start, versus being buried in thoughts, beliefs, or fears about your entire project or task. If you can do one small thing each day in the direction of your larger, more important tasks, and when you can put a big check beside these high-value undertakings, you'll find that your entire day feels more satisfying than any amount of random and distracting busyness or internet scrolling can ever provide.

ADHD-Friendly Quick Summary

- The true source of procrastination for adults with ADHD is overwhelm.
- Overwhelm causes us to freeze. When we don't know how to start something, it keeps us in stall mode.
- To overcome procrastination, you need to use simple tools that will work with your ADHD brain: use verbs to give energy to your calendar items, set your own limits, remember your Big Why, and if you're a perfectionist, aim for 90 percent (which is excellent by any standard!).
- Interrupt your distractions: Add emotional words to your digital reminders and messages, and schedule emails to send to yourself to get back on task.

ONE FOCUS

Five-Minute Freedom Schedule

Choose one goal or task that you've been procrastinating on. For one week, write in your calendar when you will spend five minutes each day taking a tiny action step toward completing it. These five minutes are nonnegotiable. You may find that these five minutes are more productive in the morning, or you can schedule them in the evening. Either way, it should be at a consistent time throughout the week if possible (e.g., five minutes every day anytime between 9:00 and 10:00 p.m.). Spending these five minutes each day will get you started and moving forward.

At the end of the week, record all the progress you've made in your notebook and notice how much closer you are now compared to only a week ago.

20

Stay on Track and Follow Through

Imagine if, whenever you found yourself lost in thought, drifting down a deep rabbit hole far away from your intended task, there was a magic button you could press to catapult you out of the hole and back to whatever you were initially doing. There actually kind of is—really! For those of us prone to losing hours (or years) of productivity to derailment and daydreams, you can leverage your brain's love of stimulus and use it for good. When you incorporate something that's highly engaging with a less engaging task, you can stay focused and get back on track more easily. It's like pressing your brain's ON switch.

☑ STATE CHANGES: WAKING UP YOUR BRAIN

We all have three states—mental (what we are thinking), emotional (how we are feeling), and physical (what we are doing), and all three are interconnected! For example, when you *think* about a terrible loss, you *feel* sad, and your body *responds* physically as well: your gaze lowers, your body posture curves forward, and your eyes may even tear up. This is an example of how all three of our states are connected to each other; and the amazing thing is that by changing one state, you can change them all! So let's say that you want to eventually change your emotional state (one of the hardest states to change), or you're losing your concentration and want to "press your brain's ON switch" to get back to what you were doing. Which of your states is the fastest and easiest to change in order to change them all?

I'll give you one guess . . .

It's your physical state.

Because all three states are connected, when you change your physical state, your mental and emotional state will automatically follow as quickly as if you've pushed a button! You can make a simple change to your physical state for as little as thirty seconds to three minutes—anything from drinking a glass of ice-cold lemon water, to a bit of physical exercise, to singing a song out loud. Almost instantly, your brain becomes more engaged, and you can go back to what you were doing recharged and refreshed. This not only helps with concentration but also with mood management—really anything that's impacted by your tendency to get absorbed by emotional or intellectual distractions.

When you change your physical state, your mental and emotional state will automatically follow.

Think of it as a friendly wake-up call for your brain comparable to splashing cold water on your face (which technically also works).

Here are a few examples of our clients' favorite state changes for you to use when you need a quick brain refresh to get back on track—or for when you want to change a mood that's not working for you at the moment:

☑ Top 15 List of Awesome State Changes

- Go outside without your phone for a two-minute walk (bonus if it's a cold day). Or simply sit outside for a couple of minutes and enjoy the fresh air.
- Do any physical exercise in *ultraslow* motion for two minutes, like three slow-motion burpees or ten slow-motion wall push-ups.
- Engage in mindfulness exercises: try focusing on your breath, taking a meditation walk, or simply noticing for one minute what "is" around you.
- Stand up and run in place for thirty seconds.
- Door Slaps: reconnect with your ten-year-old self by going around your home and jumping to slap the top of as many doorways as you can in one minute.
- Sing! It is nearly impossible to feel anxious, upset, or frustrated if you're singing your favorite song out loud.
- If you're home, brush your teeth and gargle with strong/minty mouthwash.
- Walk or run up and down a flight of stairs three or four times.
- Engage in a two-minute speed-clean, a.k.a. the Two-Minute Tidy, with your favorite high-energy music playing.

(continued on next page)

(continued from previous page)

- Have a menthol throat lozenge or mint and drink a glass of cold water immediately after.
- Find your favorite comedian online and watch for two to five minutes while standing up—*purposely* smile or laugh out loud when you hear something funny. (Set a timer. Don't get lost in watching!)
- Eat an apple (or a fruit of your choice) veeeery s-l-o-w-l-y. Notice its flavor, texture, and so on.
- If you're home, take a coolish two-minute shower.
- Turn on your favorite music and move your body or dance for an entire song.
- Balance on one leg for as long as you can while reading something or checking your emails.

State changes are one of the simplest tools an ADHDer can use in many situations to stay on track, elevate their mood, and improve productivity. All these state-change techniques will engage your brain through your body, but there are other ways you can kick your brain into gear to become more focused.

☑ MAKING IT FUN: GAMIFYING

You've probably read lots of tips about getting things done, and they may not have worked for you because they didn't fully tap into your brain's need for things to be interesting in order to stick with it and get them done.

Gamifying can turn anything you need to do, especially repetitive tasks, into a fun activity. When you have ADHD, "make it fun so you can get it done." We talked about this concept in chapter 17 with making organization strategies as entertaining as possible, and those exact same strategies can be applied here and in other areas of your life as well. You can use gamifying to stay on track with almost anything.

Zoe—Playing Her Version of Beat the Clock

Zoe works for an accountant, and tax time is a major stressor, but it is also incredibly tedious, as it involves doing a lot of data entry. She has often found herself daydreaming during the task so much so that it takes her forever to complete it all, putting her in danger of losing her job. That was until we incorporated state changes as well as creating a mini tax-time race (or game) to help her stay on track and complete the extra-boring parts of her job on time. She looks at the material she needs to enter and then guesses how many minutes it might take her. Once she's taken a guess, she tries to beat her number. When she achieves her target time and gets her work done, she treats herself to her favorite latte.

Like Zoe, you can play your own version of beat the clock and try to get a task done in under a certain amount of time. Or if it is something that you do every day—your morning routine, for example—keep track of how long it takes you, and then see if you can beat your time from one day to the next.

☑ Dice Roll

This is a favorite of so many of our clients. If you're losing your focus and want to refresh with a physical state change, make it more interesting by adding spontaneity and surprise. Roll one or two or more dice to determine your next state change (e.g., rolling a 2 = ninety seconds of slow-motion burpees; rolling a 10 = suck on a breath mint followed by drinking a glass of cold water, etc.). You'll first want to make a sheet with a legend that tells you what you'll be doing with each dice roll so you won't need to think about it at the time. The more dice you play with, the more options you can have. For example, here's a legend if you only have one die with just six options:

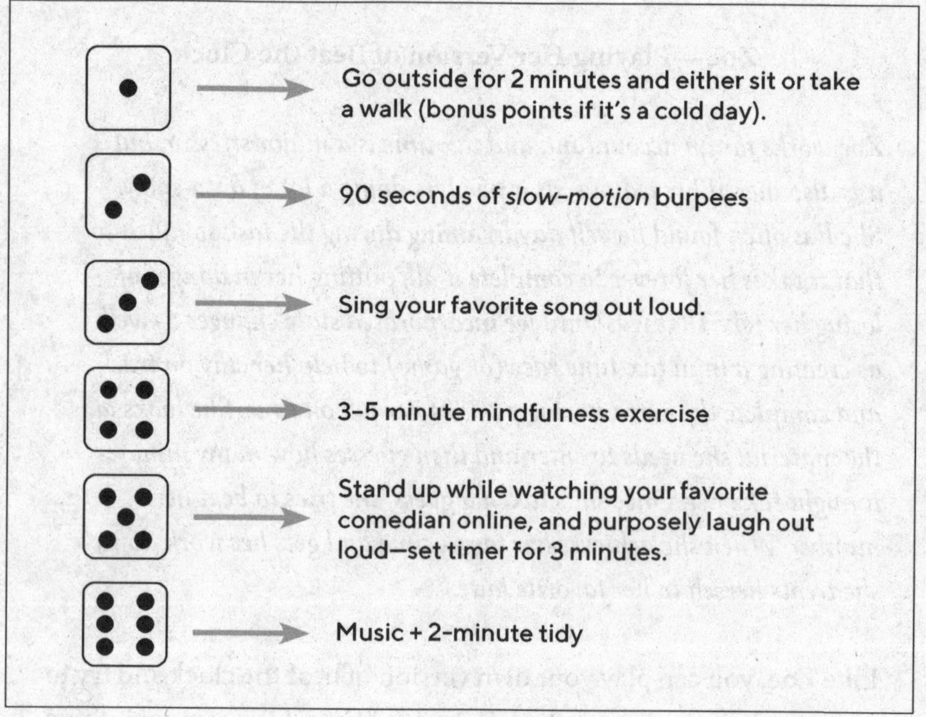

☑ Time Blasts

Beyond using Time Blasts to get more organized, a timer can be an effective tool for getting reengaged and refocused on anything you are trying to accomplish. For tasks that take a long time, if you find yourself drifting, set a timer for ten or fifteen minutes. Every ten- or fifteen-minute round is a Time Blast. The point is to see how much you can get done in a small amount of time (a Time Blast) or, conversely, how many Time Blasts it takes you to complete certain activities.

☑ Points System

Accumulating points and trying to get a high score motivated us as children; it works for practically every video game player in existence, and it'll help motivate you now, too! Assign points to all your to-do list items according to what you perceive their value to be. This will significantly help with prioritizing your tasks as well if you want to limit your to-do list to three items at a time, as we discussed in chapter 16.

Low Value (nonessential tasks, but we do them anyway): replying to low-priority emails, excessive research, organizing computer files that we rarely use = 2 points.

Medium Value (essential but nonurgent tasks): networking, routine housework, scheduling appointments, conducting progress meetings with team members, grocery shopping, general administrative work = 10 points.

High Value (essential tasks with a direct impact on your goals and overall success): completing critical work projects, exercise, nurturing important personal relationships, key research, financial management, quality family time = 20 points.

To up the ante, feel free to create a rule that will allow you to add bonus points. For example, if you complete the top three items on your to-do list, give yourself twenty bonus points. Or if you complete one of your highest-value tasks before lunch, you earn thirty bonus points. You can create a weekly goal for how many points you will try to score. Total your points at the end of the week, and try to beat your score each week! Reward yourself for earning a certain number of points in a day or beating your score from the previous week.

If you want to raise the stakes even more, you can create a competition between yourself and a friend. The person with the most points gets a reward of their choice.

These are all effective ways to wake up your brain when you're distracted and bored, and bring it back to whatever you need to be doing.

HIJACKED BY SIDETRACKS (A.K.A. NOT FOLLOWING THROUGH)

Beyond getting sidetracked in the moment, there's an even bigger challenge that many of us face: getting sidetracked for years at a time, or possibly for our entire lives.

Picture this: You're watching a major track-and-field event where, halfway through a race, one of the runners looks over to the side, turns, and immediately runs off the track, dashes up into the stands, makes a beeline for the snack bar, grabs something delicious, then bolts out of the stadium. And then, unbelievably, that same runner continues sprinting at full speed to a different track at another stadium to join another race, only to repeat the process—dashing off the track, heading to the stands, then the snack bar, but this time for some ice cream, and then she's off to yet another track . . . This bizarre routine persists for a staggering *thirty-five years* or more!

That exhausted runner is an outstanding athlete, maybe one of the best ever; yet she never gets to win, or even *finish*, a single race! But she did get to eat a lot of different snack bar snacks, which were pretty good, so there's that.

This routine may feel familiar to those of us who habitually start things with enthusiasm but then struggle to follow through on them. Maybe you got involved in a relationship that was off-the-charts incredible at the beginning, but when things started to become routine, you felt the need to bail. Or maybe you wanted to earn a particular academic degree at college, but the hours and hours of studying got the best of you. You may have started a new job (or three or ten) that sounded great when you applied but grew tedious after the first few months, so you moved on. Or you really wanted to join an in-person book club, knowing you're desperate for some live social interaction; yet despite enjoying the first meeting, you never went back again.

It seems like there is *always* something else that grabs your attention. Over there is a different idea, a new initiative, maybe a different health regimen that promises to be so much easier and more effective than the last one! This new idea is extremely fun and exciting! With absolutely no obstacles in sight. Before you know it, it's buh-bye to goal #1 and helloooo to goal #2.

You go from idea to idea, chasing down anything that is new, exciting, compelling, and *definitely* something you're going to do, leaving in your wake dozens and dozens of unrealized inspirations. It's like you've created an entire cemetery filled with good ideas that never came to fruition. One of my clients expressed this reality so poignantly.

"I had so many dreams, I call it Land of the Broken Dreams, where you see these 'could be' dreams that I never worked on and were just left there to rot and die. And as I go through my house, I see little piles of broken dreams everywhere..."

Ultimately, very few sidetracks are as interesting on the second day as they were on the first, and yet you keep chasing them, or hop from one to another for decades of your life. You're always looking for fulfillment in the novelty of something brand-new, going down a path you never meant to follow until one day you realize that you are in a city, a career, or a relationship that you never intended or wanted to be in. Ever! An innocent distraction has become your day-to-day reality.

Feelings of potential loss become overshadowed by the intense high and exhilaration of moving on to the next new thing.

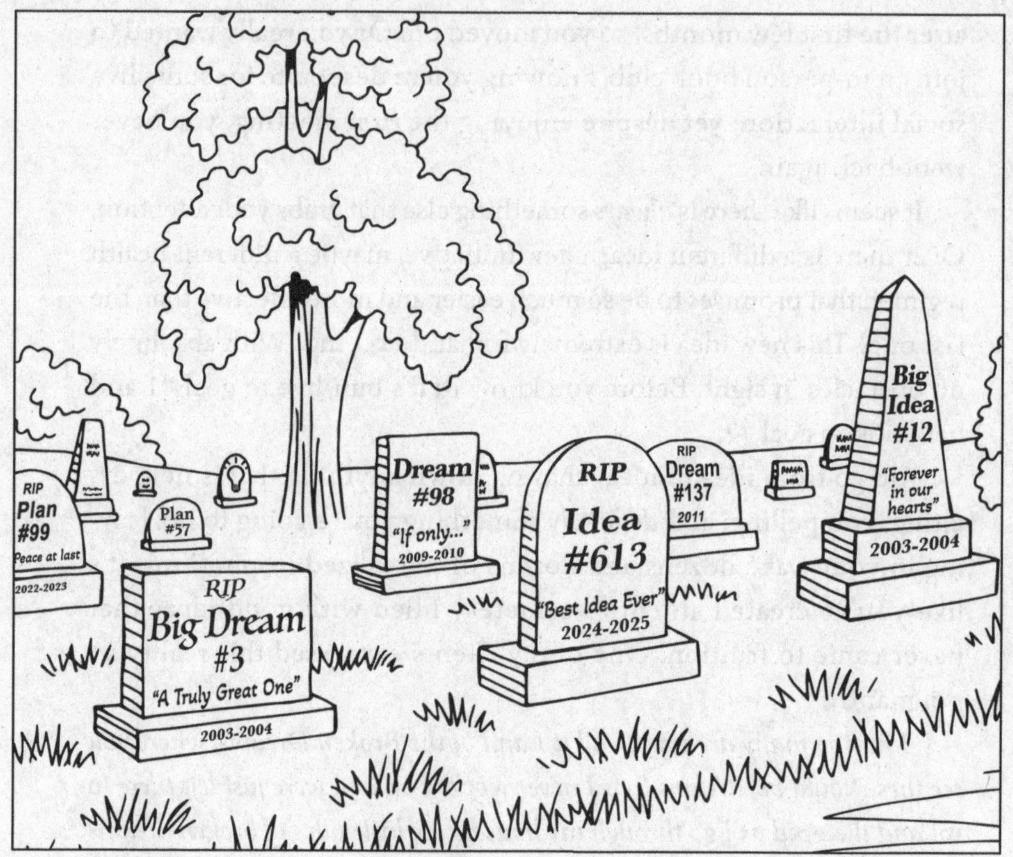

The Cemetery of Broken Dreams

If you recognize this pattern in your own life, you are not alone. ADHDers have a chronic challenge with following through on what we start. I've worked with so many people over the age of seventy who feel they've never accomplished anything meaningful in their lives. It's so sad, because although they have achievements to be proud of, when they look back, they are more likely to recall and regret the things they didn't follow through on, when any feelings of loss they may have felt at the time were overshadowed by the intense high and exhilaration of moving on to the next new thing.

CROSSING THE FINISH LINE: HOW TO FOLLOW THROUGH

Undoubtedly, there will be times when we know we must switch from one thing to another, and sometimes it can work out amazingly well, which is great! The problem arises when you realize that your life has become a never-ending cycle of starting, stopping, and turning around, which is common for women with ADHD. We get caught up in "life," and for so many of us, "being busy being busy" is our happy place—we're pulled in so many directions, constantly engaged with work, entertainment, leisure activities, groups we felt obliged to join, and all the things that fill up our days that simultaneously keep us from sticking with a path that's more meaningful for us.

☑ Connect Follow-Through to Your Big Why

Some of the most effective follow-through strategies that have helped our clients stick with their intentions have involved helping them reconnect with the reasons that pushed them to pursue their initial path in the first place. Just as we previously talked about how connecting our goals to a Big Why makes them juicy, meaningful, and emotionally resonant, we can use the same principle to help you get back on track and follow through, even if you've been caught up in a sidetrack.

When we're impulsively escaping boredom and seeking stimulus by going from one thing to the next, we inevitably miss opportunities. This happens to all of us. Let's consider what could happen if we tie a "lost" opportunity to our Big Why:

1. Take out your notebook and write down something meaningful that you said you wanted to do and had already put in motion (yes!) but stopped making progress somewhere along the way.

It can be as big or as small as you like. For example:

* Starting a side gig to make extra money. You even drafted your website!
* Planning a much-needed weekend getaway with your friends. You even chose the weekend *and* the location.
* Learning how to ________. You already signed up for the free trial of the course!

2. Now, connect whatever you most recently didn't follow through with (that you'd still like to do) to a Big Why by asking yourself these questions and writing down your answers in your notebook:
   * How will I feel once I've finally accomplished this?
   * What other possibilities will open up once I've followed through with this?
   * How might specific people in my life think about me if I follow through with this?
   * How will *I* feel about myself after finishing this?

The more you get emotionally tied to the different possibilities of following through with what you said you'd do, the more your brain will pull you toward actually following through with it.

☑ Replace Your Nonurgent Commitments

Do social and nonurgent commitments fill up your entire life? Are you staying in busy mode because you're afraid you'll lose your momentum, or feel bored, or maybe there are painful emotions, or a difficult situation that you're trying to distract yourself from? Maybe you are letting other people influence what is "urgent" and you are taking on their problems? Before you commit to jumping into something else, ask what is driving your decision. Notice when you are "being busy being busy," rather than following through with what's more important for you.

Here's a quick challenge: Think about one time-filler activity that you often do, then choose *not* to do it for three days. Common examples are playing games on your phone, binge-watching shows, and online browsing.

Now, **replace** that activity with something constructive that you know will move you toward *anything* more meaningful that you have pushed aside.

Even if you replace *less than half* of the time you spend on the time-filler activity, after just a few days, you'll notice a difference in how far you've moved toward following through on your objectives! One of my clients who habitually watched two hours of TV each evening before bed decided to replace the first thirty minutes to go back to learning guitar, something she had wanted to get back into for *decades* but hadn't made time for. It's taken a while, but now she's at the point where it's become her favorite thing to do and she's even writing her own songs.

Notice when you are "being busy being busy," rather than following through with what's more important for you.

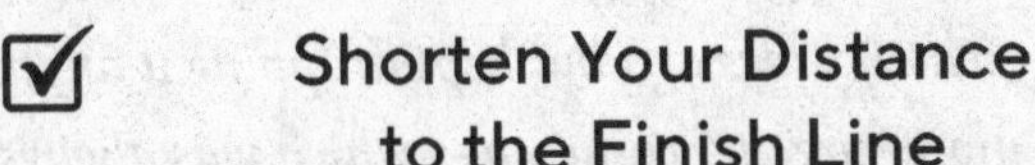

Shorten Your Distance to the Finish Line

You can't win a race if you stop before the finish line. If you think of completing a task like it's a race that you intend to win, it's more difficult to go off course in the middle, even if there is a *very* compelling sidetrack that wants to pull you away. One way to get across the finish line and get the "win" without being distracted by something else is by moving the finish line closer to you! This can be achieved by dividing your big goals into smaller, incremental goals. We have talked about this previously (and we may do so again), but it's worth repeating. When each small step becomes a goal in and of itself, those small goals will build toward your larger goal.

You can't win a race if you stop before the finish line.

For example, if you want to lose weight, first focus on elevating your heart rate for a full five minutes each day, or replace one junk food item a day with something healthy that also tastes good. If you want to start your own business, first focus on getting just one paying customer or making your first hundred dollars, or simply writing out a short, first draft of a business plan. You can master the art of following through by successfully completing very small goals, one after another. This builds momentum, instills a natural desire to keep "winning," boosts your self-esteem, and makes it much easier to follow through and finish whatever you start.

Dawn—Getting to Vacation Step-by-Step

Dawn is a very busy mom who had been planning a trip to Disney for the last ten (!) years, but she couldn't seem to make it happen. When we first met, her kids were eleven and thirteen, yet at the rate she'd been going, her kids would have been married with kids of their own by the time they finally got to see Mickey Mouse. She started doing the research years ago but kept dropping it anytime something slightly more "urgent" came up—which was always. She'd then beat herself up thinking there was something wrong with her because she didn't get it all done.

For her to get some perspective, we worked on her initial intention for this trip and why she wanted to bring her family to Disney in the first place. We then looked at all the things that she did every day and what had been taking her off this path. We began to move the finish line closer to her by creating smaller wins every week that she could achieve—first setting dates, next booking flights, and so on. Each of those steps had smaller steps within them (checking the kids' school calendars, finding her travel points account), and she wasn't allowed to stop working on any of these smaller steps until it was complete, so she was creating a path of small yet important completions on the way to Disney.

It felt like it was taking forever, but from the time we started working on this trip to when they got on the plane was only four months, which was a huge improvement over the ten years she had been thinking about it! Now when she looks at the family photos from their incredible trip, she knows not only that she can complete what she starts but also that she can likely do it again in the future.

☑ Building Your Follow-Through Muscle

To get into the new habit of finishing what you start, you need to start small with those "little things that you wanted to finish but didn't" tasks.

Each day, take two to three minutes to complete only *one* of those small things. For example: Finish paying a bill, finish washing the dishes that are still in the sink (time yourself!), make one appointment you intended to make but haven't made yet (you know the one I mean), complete the next step of a big work task that you got distracted from, call back the person whose conversation got cut short because you had to go, or finish reading this chapter all the way to the end (you're almost there).

The point is to get yourself into the follow-through habit! After each completion, write down in your notebook what it was that you successfully finished. At the end of a few days, look at all the little things you ended up completing to prove to yourself that, yes, you actually *do* follow through on what you start.

Every time you complete any small task, you are sending your brain a powerful message that says, "See, I said I was going to do this one little thing, and I *did* it!" When you're conscious of noting each small completion for a few days, you will absolutely notice a change for the better in how you follow through on bigger things until it becomes the habitual way that you do things more often than not.

Look at all the little things you ended up completing to prove to yourself that, yes, you actually *do* follow through on what you start.

ADHD-Friendly Quick Summary

- The quickest way to get out of your head is to get into your body. Use physical state changes to wake up your brain, boost your mood, become more focused, and increase productivity.
- Gamify repetitive tasks by using Time Blasts and points systems. Try anything that inspires you to stay engaged.
- To help you stay on track and follow through, connect what you want to finish to your Big Why. Think about how you will feel once it's completed.
- Think of one time-filler activity that you can easily replace—or partially replace—with a task that helps you follow through on something much more meaningful.
- Move the finish line closer to you! Get in the habit of following through and finishing very small steps. Note each of your completions and own the fact that you're someone who can follow through!

ONE FOCUS

Physical State Change to Stay on Track and Get Stuff Done

Come up with three or four go-to physical state change activities that would be easy for you to implement (eat something healthy in super-slow motion, brush your teeth, go outside *without* your phone and breathe in fresh air for two minutes—even if it's freezing cold!—jog in place for ninety seconds, crank up the music and dance) and write them down in your notebook.

Each day for one week, put any one of your state change activities into action when you:

- start to lose your focus while you're trying to work, or
- want to elevate your mood, or
- need to finish a boring task that you don't want to do (like dishes, emails, laundry, paperwork, and so on).

Once you get in the habit of incorporating simple and engaging physical state changes throughout your day, you'll begin doing them automatically and will soon notice how much more focused and productive you feel on a regular basis.

21

Optimize Your Memory

Do people ever get upset with you or call you absent-minded or inconsiderate because you're forgetful? Are you critical of *yourself* because you're forgetful, thinking, *Wow, I'm the worst friend—I forgot her birthday, and it was a week ago!* Or *How did I forget that I made plans with them for Saturday—what is wrong with me!?* Have you ever tried extra hard to remember something, even repeating it a dozen times to yourself, only to forget what you were trying to remember five minutes later? Are you concerned that any memory issues you have now will get worse as you get older?

In general, people with ADHD have challenges with short-term memory and can easily forget the things that are important to them and the people they care about, but it's *not* because you don't care or that you have a subpar brain. The reason information doesn't stick with you is a reflection of the way your brain *insists* on processing 1,001 things all at the same time.

For example, I tend to forget anything and everything that comes to me while I'm picking my kids up from school. I never understood why my memory seemed to shut down during pickup time until I took a closer look at what was going on. I realized that when I'm at my desk working (basically doing one thing), I'm thinking about what I'm looking at on my computer, and I can easily write down whatever I want to remember for later (remember the Parking Lot?). When I'm alone in my car at school pickup waiting for my kids, I tend to think about:

- My children's whereabouts.
- Who's singing the song coming through my car speakers right now.
- If I should ask my son how he did on his test or wait for him to tell me.
- Where I need to take my kids after school, what time they need to be there, and how much traffic I'll hit on the way.
- Where I can find a sweater like the one that mom standing over there is wearing.
- What we should have for dinner tonight.
- What's in the unread messages that pinged on my phone while I was driving.
- Those three work situations that I need to figure out by tomorrow.

With all that information buzzing around in the exact same place in my head at the same time, what does my ADHD brain naturally prioritize? You guessed it—the thing that has the greatest amount of stimulus and interest attached to it. For me, that would either be where I could find that same sweater before I never see it again or planning that night's dinner, but it would be different for all of us. So, while waiting in the pickup line, you might:

- Look for a parking spot so you can get out to find your kids because you still can't see them.
- Find out who's singing that song on the radio.
- Quickly look up the appropriate level of parental involvement regarding a sixth grader's test scores.
- Look up simple dinner recipes.
- Figure out the most prominent features of that mom's sweater to look into later.
- Reply to one of those messages that came in while you were driving.
- None of the above, because seventeen new thoughts just flew into your brain in the last five seconds, and you want to focus on one of those.

The reason information doesn't stick with you is a reflection of the way your brain *insists* on processing 1,001 things all at the same time.

It's very hard to remember something—even if it's important—when there are a hundred other things competing for your attention. Imagine your thoughts are like a classroom full of young children. I'm sure you've noticed that, typically, the "problem kid" gets most of the teacher's time and attention, while there are twenty-five or more other kids in the class who also need attention. That is what's happening in your brain with all your thoughts at any given time—the most high-impact or disruptive thoughts get the attention—your *brain's* attention, not *your* attention.

So, contrary to what you may have always thought about yourself, you likely don't have a "bad" memory. You just have too many things that are simultaneously vying for your attention to let just one idea be front and center.

Memory issues can take their biggest toll on important relationships for ADHDers, because the things that your heart registers as important are not always the same things that stimulate your memory. In relationships, it's the little things that matter most, and those little things are exactly what the ADHD brain has the tendency to overlook. That's why your child can remind you that their big game is on Friday at 3:30 p.m., and you can promise them that you'll be there, but when the day arrives you're a no-show because you're trying to get something critical done at work. There's nothing you wanted more than to be cheering in the stands, but because your brain didn't put urgency on that information, it was completely obliterated by the thoughts that were louder and more alarming.

At the extreme end, friendships, romances, and even families can fall apart because of the tendency of the ADHD brain to prioritize only things that stimulate it—both the positives and the negatives. However, because your brain is awesome at remembering what it finds interesting, you can tap into this skill to improve your ability to make things stick in your mind.

MAKE IT INTERESTING TO MAKE IT MEMORABLE

To make anything more memorable, create a visual image with a strong sensation or emotion attached to it.

Here are some strategies for using mnemonic devices like imagery, emotion, and even your senses to help tap into your ability to remember what's most interesting.

Link to Something Visual

Our ability to recall visuals is *much* stronger than it is for words. To make anything more memorable, create a visual image with a strong sensation or emotion attached to it.

☑ ***Words:*** Let's say you're trying to learn Chinese, and you can't remember the word for *hello*. Well, the word is *nǐ hǎo*, pronounced "knee how." Visualize yourself in detail walking into your favorite Chinese restaurant (can you see it?), and as you're about to say hello to the hostess, you trip and bang your knee hard against the floor (ow!). Picture the scenario: How did you bang your knee? What color was the floor? What would you say? "Knee (h)ow!" Imagine you're on the floor holding your knee, and in your mind, say it again.

☑ ***Names:*** Focus on the person you're meeting while purposefully turning down the volume of distracting background noise in your mind about where you've seen them before, what they do, and so on. To help create a visual to remember their name, picture yourself writing their name three times on a wall in huge letters, in a color of spray paint that matches their personality.

You can also match names to an image so they will be easier to recall.

Abby = abracadabra (Abby's now a magician wearing a top hat); Sandy = beach (imagine Sandy at the beach or covered with sand). Basically, transform them and their name into something more colorful, interesting, and memorable. You can choose a single facial feature of theirs, like a tiny nose, or an eyebrow ring, or a goatee, or a receding hairline, or a dimple that stands out to you, and connect it with their name, like "Prachi with the dimple," which may be easier to remember than just "Prachi." Another tip is to say their name once again when you say goodbye to further lock it in your mind. You can also type or record their name into a note on your phone, then at the end of the day, go over those notes, so the name of the new person ends up going into your long-term memory.

Engage Your Senses

"The more senses that are engaged, the more attention the brain pays." See it. Hear it. Physically touch or move with it if you have to!

☑ ***Sight*:** In the same way that creating a visual helps you make connections with names and other languages, you can create a high-stimulus visual of anything you want to remember. Always losing your car keys? Next time you put them down, imagine that they have exploded in the place you've put them and are engulfed in a raging fire. Sound a little extreme? It is, but the next time you think of your keys, you'll remember that dramatic image and be able to find them.

☑ ***Sound*:** Say whatever you are trying to remember *out loud* and repeat it a few times. Vocalizing it forces you to slow down and organize your thoughts. What's more, hearing the words as you think them has a "dual encoding" effect that makes the memory more likely to stick. You're speaking the information *and* you're hearing it. This is also a great way for ADHDers to study—read your notes out loud into a voice memo, and then play it back so you can listen to what you have just read.

☑ ***Sing It*:** Singing to memorize information can work quite well—just think of all the kids across generations who have sung the ABC song to learn the alphabet! A good beat and tune will stimulate your brain's ability to remember, so replace a song's lyrics with the information you are trying to remember and sing it! I started using this method to memorize multiplication tables in third grade, and I still use it to this day anytime I need to remember something specific.

☑ ***Movement/Touch*:** This technique is great for kinesthetic learners (i.e., people who learn best by feeling and doing, as opposed to by hearing or seeing). As you're trying to encode the information into your brain, engage in a physical activity. This can be as simple as taking a walk or pumping your legs on a park swing while listening to the notes you just recorded on your phone. When I was in university (pre-smartphone days) I used to study for my final exams by taking my textbooks and highlighters to the university fitness center and putting them on the magazine holder that was attached to the treadmill or exercise bike. The harder I exercised, the easier it was to highlight key points, and the better I was able to remember everything I was reading. It was like my leg work was physically pushing the information into my brain. Sure, I felt incredibly self-conscious being the *only* person in our super-crowded gym with a textbook (most people had sports or fashion magazines propped on their equipment), but I'm positive it's one of the main reasons I was able to graduate.

The more senses that are engaged, the more attention the brain pays.

All these methods force you to become much more present and attentive, while at the same time creating a form of stimulus. Beyond improving your memory, adding an extra spoonful of interest in whatever way works for you gets your brain to pay closer attention.

☑ YOUR BACKUP MEMORY

There are some things that you need to remember that simply can't be made more interesting no matter what you do. Also, there are things you need to remember that you really don't want to think about. Luckily, the tools we've already discussed in earlier chapters (remember?) will help you keep track of the things you *don't* want taking up precious space in your beautiful mind.

***Extended Parking Lot*:** One of your time management tools in chapter 18 is to have a Parking Lot to manage distracting thoughts, and you can use this as a memory tool as well. Many of our clients are in the habit of keeping their Parking Lot notepad nearby at all times (even in the car) so they can write down thoughts and ideas that pop up while they are doing something else that they want to remember later.

***Calendar*:** Hopefully by now, you're actively using a calendar. Get in the habit of using it consistently and it will serve as your backup memory for *everything* in your life that has a time and date associated with it.

***Alarms*:** This is especially useful for tasks that aren't part of your regular routine—like appointments or meetings. Set one alarm for the day before as a reminder, and a second alarm for an hour beforehand. When the second alarm sounds, if commuting isn't required, reset it for fifty minutes later (or adjust as needed for preparation time) to give yourself a final prompt to make sure you're fully ready. This way, if you become totally immersed in something else, you're still less likely to forget—especially if you snooze it to go off again in eight minutes.

***Phone Memos and Reminders*:** You can get in the habit of putting ideas or lists on your phone apps as well. Shopping lists, books or movies you hear about, sporting events, concerts, travel locations, and so on. Once you enter it in, it remains, and then you just need to remember to check the app on your phone.

Forgetting and missing important events or absent-mindedly hurting the feelings of people you love no longer has to be part of your modus operandi. You have the ability to do the thing you said you'd do, show up when you say you will, come through when you said you would, be a good friend, and do many of the things made easier with a good memory. All you have to *remember* is to intentionally infuse whatever you want to remember with extra mental stimulus and energy.

ADHD-Friendly Quick Summary

- You likely don't have a bad memory but rather a brain that tends to remember what's most compelling.
- Instead of letting any interesting thought clamor for your attention, purposefully choose to make your important thoughts stimulating and memorable.
- Make things memorable by making them more interesting: Connect names, words, or ideas to something visual. Say things out loud so that you're speaking it *and* hearing it simultaneously.
- Pair what you need to remember with physical activity to stimulate your brain so that it can pay attention more easily.
- Use tools like an extended Parking Lot, your calendar, alarms, and phone memos to serve as your backup memory.

ONE FOCUS

Using Tangible Visuals!

Visuals are a fantastic way to keep something front and center in your mind. For one week, pick one thing for each day that you need to remember to do (that you tend to forget because they are routine or boring). For example, mundane activities like grocery shopping, laundry, submitting work projects on time, making a doctor's appointment, tracking your spending, and so on will often need a little something extra to make them stand out enough for you to remember them.

Choose a tangible, hard-copy (screen-free) visual for each task (*not* a sticky note if you already have sticky notes that you consistently ignore all over the place). Put the tangible visual where you'll see it to make sure you remember to do the task. These visuals will be incredibly helpful in triggering your memory. For example:

- Grocery shopping bag hung on your door to remind you to pick up food.
- One smelly sock on your doorknob. (Really, to remind you to do laundry! Not surprisingly, this one works fast.)
- Photos next to your computer (a home-printed picture of your kid in their sports uniform with a note that has their upcoming game time written on it).
- Your guitar propped in a prominent place in the room where you spend the most time (to remind you to play *and* practice).
- A handwritten list of work projects (and names of others collaborating with you) and what your main goal for each project is!

Whichever items you choose, make sure it's something that will trigger your memory and not just become physical clutter. Implement this strategy for at least two things you need to remember to do this week and watch how they become more sticky in your mind.

22

Communicate Effectively and Be Understood

Communication is an essential aspect of human interaction that goes far beyond the exchange of words. It's how we share our thoughts, emotions, ideas, and experiences. We draw on our communication to establish connections, build relationships, and shape the way we're perceived and understood by others, which contributes to our impact on the world. Yet for people with ADHD, our communications are heavily affected by some of our most common challenges—like impulsivity and emotional dysregulation, often resulting in misunderstandings with friends, family, employers, colleagues, and nearly every human we interact with.

By improving your communication skills, you can strengthen your relationships, further your personal and professional goals, and leave a positive impression on others. Life will feel less stressful and upsetting, and you'll be in fewer situations trying to explain yourself after being completely misunderstood (again).

COMMUNICATION CHALLENGES

If you notice that communication is a challenge for you, or if others tell you that it is, or if you get overwhelmed when needing to communicate something important and you never seem to know what to say or how to say it, you're in excellent company. See if any of these common communication challenges hit home:

- ***Speaking in circles*****:** Having difficulty getting to the point.

- ***Oversharing and letting it allll come out*****:** Difficulty organizing and prioritizing your thoughts so that your communication comes out as a long stream of consciousness.

- ***No filter*****:** Because your mind is going so fast, slowing down to read verbal and nonverbal cues from others is difficult, so you impulsively say whatever you think in the moment, whether or not it's appropriate.

- ***Second-guessing yourself*****:** You are so preoccupied wondering what to say and when that your mind pulls you out of the conversation, and you're left with very few words. This is the exact opposite of having "no filter."

- ***Interrupting and blurting out*****:** Your brain may jump ahead to the end of what you think the other person's point is before they have finished speaking, prompting you to blurt out thoughts about what you *assume* they're going to say before you lose the thought.

- ***Missing what others are saying*****:** You may have trouble hearing others because you are listening so intently to your own thoughts while the other person is talking.

- ***Being too intense*****:** When expressing yourself, you may be overly enthusiastic, expressive, loud, or emotional. Your intensity and emotionality can push others away.

- ***Being overly confrontational*****:** You argue out of habit, to prove yourself or because you simply need to be acknowledged as being right, and usually, you don't recognize that you are doing it or that it is a problem.

- ***Being overly sensitive*****:** You may take what others say much too personally (even constructive criticism) and lose the ability to be objective.

- ***Repeating yourself*****:** You may repeat yourself or say something in multiple ways because you anticipate that you will be misunderstood.

- ***Trying for perfection*****:** When engaging in written communication, you may devote hours to crafting the perfect email, constantly second-guessing if what you are writing is correct or valid.

Poor communication skills can culminate in extreme loneliness, job instability, relationship turmoil, and feeling generally disconnected from others. Some women with ADHD feel perpetually misunderstood by everyone around them, even their closest family members. When people don't advance in their careers, or lose their jobs, it's not always because they can't master the day-to-day job requirements. They can be pretty good at the actual "work" involved, yet can also be considered "difficult to work with," which can mean a lot of different things. Maybe their attitude comes off as unprofessional. Maybe they have a hard time complying with procedures. Or they speak impulsively. Maybe they have a hard time getting along with others, or they've received multiple notices or warnings and don't know how to correct their behavior. In many cases, these aren't unqualified people or lazy workers. They're almost always intelligent, well-meaning people with excellent skills and intentions who haven't yet learned how to communicate well.

At the end of the day, our capacity to listen and how we respond to others is going to have a huge influence on our relationships and how we move forward in our lives.

LISTENING TO COMMUNICATE

We have two ears and one mouth so that we can listen twice as much as we speak.

—Epictetus

One key skill can help you to become an excellent communicator: listening.

Have you ever found yourself in a conversation where, just as you finish saying something that was important to you, the person you were speaking to responds with a blank stare, followed by "Mm-hmm—yeah, totally," before disconnecting from the conversation? That person obviously wasn't listening. Do you remember how you felt at that moment? Or, worse—maybe *you* were not listening, and they flatly informed you, "I literally just said that." You may have been told repeatedly by your close friends and family, or maybe your exes, that you're not the best listener. And if you have ADHD, chances are they're right. That can make things challenging because listening is the most important element of communication.

When you listen, people feel respected, recognized, and validated. As you can probably imagine, people are usually attracted to someone who connects with them and makes them feel heard. Look at some of the most magnetic leaders in the world and study their style—you'll notice that when they interact with people, they appear to be totally present and in the moment. They're not looking around the room or interrupting to interject their own views. They're totally focused on the other person, nodding, and (when appropriate) asking questions that will further the conversation. They behave as if there's nothing they'd rather be doing than hearing what the other person has to say. And the person who's being listened to feels totally heard and seen.

Listening is the most important element of communication.

Think about (or imagine) the last time somebody was listening to you that way and how *you* felt. Some of my clients have even connected an experience of being listened to so intently with a time that they've fallen in love! It can be that powerful.

Are You Going to Explode?

When others talk, you might initially be interested in what they're saying, but then a thought pops into your head. It could be something funny, something smart, or something that you *need* to share because you're sure you're going to forget it if you have to hold it in much longer. As soon as the other person pauses for breath, this brilliant (and urgent) response explodes out of you like soda from a shaken-up bottle.

Sometimes, your brilliant (and urgent) thought might not even wait for the other person to pause, and instead, you unintentionally burst into the middle of their sentence! You may see the speaker's raised eyebrows and feel their annoyance, but you just can't stop until your thought is set free into the world.

It can be challenging to make sense of your own thoughts, let alone everyone else's. Your thoughts are loud and intense, and it's as if you are having a conversation with two people at the same time—the person you are speaking with and the thoughts that are running through your head. There is a constant battle for your attention between what you are thinking and what the other person is saying. The conversation inside your head usually wins.

As someone with ADHD, even when you are genuinely interested in what is being said, you can find yourself thinking more about what you're going to say next than attending to what the other person is telling you, which makes it hard to listen or even to wait until you can respond in an appropriate way.

The Power of Pausing

It is impossible to fully listen to someone else while you're talking. Try it! And to be honest, staying silent for a person with ADHD is a lot harder than it is for most people. Not only is your brain moving at top speed, there's no separation between your thoughts. And let's not forget about your natural time blindness, impulsivity, impatience, and how difficult it is to wait a million hours for the other person to finish what they're saying before you can jump in.

In your heart, you're truly interested in what people around you have to say, but in reality, it's really difficult to listen attentively when your mind is filling up with nonstop, very loud, and (admit it) extremely interesting chatter.

Which brings us to a fundamental communication skill: pausing. Because it's impossible to slow down your brain (despite everyone having told you to "slow down" your entire life), many of the upcoming techniques that allow you to listen, and help others to hear and understand you, also involve ways to create three-second pauses in your communications (and in your thinking).

It might honestly feel like you're going to explode if you can't say what's on your mind right away—but you won't. You can actually press Pause on your side of the conversation without blurting out your thoughts and nothing horrible will happen—even if you totally forget what you wanted to say. The world will still spin, and the person speaking with you will enjoy the conversation that much more.

It is impossible to fully listen to someone else while you're talking.

STRATEGIES FOR BETTER COMMUNICATION

You can put these into practice right now, today, so you can become a better listener and communicator immediately. While some may not work for you, others can be extremely effective. Remember, the only strategy that is guaranteed not to work is the one that you don't try!

☑ Start Before You Speak: Set Your Intention

Think about *why* you want to communicate better in the specific situation or conversation you're about to have. Maybe you want to make a good impression, or you want to know more about another person and feel closer to them, or you're trying to avoid an argument, or you want to ask someone to do something for you, or you want to help someone you love feel understood, or *you* might just want to feel heard and understood. By communicating well, you're connecting to a bigger, more meaningful goal.

You'll want to start by creating an intention for the outcome you want. For example, when your son or daughter comes home from college for the holidays, you can repeat to yourself: *My intention with this conversation is for my child to feel totally heard and loved by me.* Once you've set that intention and continue to repeat it to yourself, the way you respond to them while you're together will be guided by that intention, and the tone will likely be much more in line with what you're going for.

When you create a strong intention for how you are going to behave, *before* the communication starts, you are *much* more likely to stay true to it.

Alternatively, you can create an intention about how you want to be seen (and heard) with your family and friends, or while you're at work. This works especially well if you find yourself interrupting people no matter who you're with. For example: *My intention is to listen to what others say, be patient, take it slow, and allow others to express themselves before I jump in.*

When you create a strong intention for how you are going to behave, *before* the communication starts, you are *much* more likely to stay true to it during the time you are engaging with someone.

☑ Get Rid of Competing Stimuli (So You Can Focus on the Person You Are Speaking With)

If you can engineer your environment to get rid of any distracting, competing stimuli, you can increase your ability to be present and engage with whomever you're speaking with. Disconnecting from distractions is great for better communication at work, but it is especially helpful if you're in a relationship or have kids. Most of us don't realize our tendency to talk to our loved ones while we're staring down at our phones.

The easiest things to eliminate are distractions like TV, your computer, and your phone. The solutions are clear: turn off the TV, close your computer or physically turn away from it, and physically move your phone out of sight—put it in a drawer, your handbag, or leave it in another room. For someone with ADHD, it's almost automatic to get laser focused on whatever is most stimulating—usually something on a screen—rather than being present with what or who is right in front of you. You may not realize that when you check your phone for what feels like only a second, you were actually looking down at it for a full minute or longer while others were talking to you. In my home, phones are not allowed at the table, and we have a designated space to put them during dinnertime so that we're not all constantly checking messages that come in during that time. It's been working (so far).

Look up from your phone, make eye contact, and connect. In fact, for the next two days, do your best to consciously make eye contact for just two or three seconds with everyone you speak with in person—colleagues, friends, your kids, your partner—and see what happens. It'll be more impactful than you might think.

Look up from your phone, make eye contact, and connect.

☑ Unload Carefully

If you tend to overshare or let everything out in a stream of consciousness, the next time you feel the urge to unload, choose one single point to discuss instead of letting them know *everything* that is on your mind. Other topics and questions will likely come up, but the other person will feel much less overwhelmed (and attacked) if you stay focused on only one point.

☑ Practice Out Loud: Role-Play

Preparing responses ahead of time and practicing them out loud can be very effective for many situations—for example, if you are often interrupted at work, you could practice saying, "I'd love to talk about this, but I'm not able to right now. Can we discuss it later?" Or you can use this in other situations when you might get emotional and impatient. Perhaps it's when you're stressed out and trying to hit a deadline? If you think of one or two standard responses, write them down, and then repeat them aloud (this is key!). You will be able to respond in a way that is more aligned with who you genuinely are rather than lashing out in a moment of high stress and frustration.

Role-playing is also helpful for everyday situations that feel awkward or when you never seem to know what to say, whether it's practicing small talk, talking with someone after they've received bad news, or asking for a raise . . . basically anytime you want to talk with someone without having your own emotions take over.

☑ Park It

If you're an impulsive speaker, which many of us are, you probably say what's on your mind as soon as it pops into your head—even if it can be hurtful, and even if it almost never works out well for you.

By choosing to park your issue until later and writing down what you're thinking, you eliminate the fear that you'll forget what you want to say while giving yourself time to regulate your emotions so that you don't say something you'll seriously regret. You can go back to it later (give it at least a night) and review what you've written, and *then* determine if it's essential that you share what you were thinking. We all know we should take the time to sleep on an angry or heated comeback, but most of us rarely do because our impulsivity takes over. If it is important to be communicated, you can decide when you are calmer the best way to phrase your words without damaging the relationship and creating resentment.

☑ Engage Your Brain

Being an attentive listener can feel like an impossible feat, no matter how hard we try. Sometimes, the person speaking is going *so* slowly that it feels like watching paint dry, and when they just can't seem to get to the point, it's torture! Sometimes it's not the delivery but the topic itself that is boring, but you know that you have to listen and contribute anyway.

There are ways to make unbearable situations like these more interesting and tolerable. Next time you are feeling distracted or catch yourself drifting off when you want to be paying attention, try these:

- Look for the speaker's purpose. What's motivating *them* to tell you this? Maybe they're trying to share something to feel respected, understood, or closer to *you*.
- Make mental notes. When you're talking with a friend or loved one, imagine there will be an exam at the end and try to take in every single thing being said as if you're going to be tested on it

later. If something gets past you, ask them to repeat it.

- If you're in a meeting, write down the main points of what you're hearing.
- Try to figure out where the person is coming from. What's interesting to them about this? Actively thinking about their perspective on a topic *versus your own opinion* about it will help you listen more attentively.

Try to take in every single thing being said as if you're going to be tested on it later.

Another way to engage your brain, as you already know, is to physically move around. For some of us, sitting still and trying to maintain eye contact can be uncomfortable and distracting, and it's nearly impossible to pay attention to anything anyone is saying if we feel physically restless. In that case, walking or pacing while in conversation can actually keep you engaged and help you stay focused on the other person. Just be sure to let them know that you're pacing *in order to listen better* or they'll think you're not paying attention.

In a videoconference, if you're not presenting and are able to turn off your video, you can move freely as long as you continue to participate so that others in the meeting will know that you're still there, and totally present with them.

☑ Avoid the Olympic-Level Long Jump . . . to Conclusions

Many of us unknowingly hijack conversations because we are certain that we know where the other person is heading, and it's not *our* fault it's taking them sooo many painful minutes to get there! In our minds, we can save everyone some time by cutting to the chase with our response. Unless, of course, we're wrong. Which we often are.

Although you may be convinced that you know what the other person is going to say, you don't. The only way to know for sure is to listen to them. To keep from jumping to conclusions too quickly, purposely shift your focus to the other person. Slow down and verify that you've understood what they are saying: "I think I get what you mean . . ." or "I hear you saying . . ."; and if you don't understand what they mean, ask a question to clarify.

Although you may be convinced that you know what the other person is going to say, you don't. The only way to know for sure is to listen to them.

Sometimes asking a question about what you just heard is the best response to what someone is saying. It forces you to press Pause on what your brain wants you to blurt out, it shows the other person that you are interested, reaffirms that what they are saying is important to you, and may help you understand something you genuinely missed (that you probably didn't notice).

☑ Turn Arguments into a Listening Game

It's helpful to remember that anytime we "win" an argument with someone, it automatically means that they "lose." How do *you* feel when someone is trying to prove you wrong? Really think about it. Do you remember how it feels when you lose to someone who insists that they're right? How do you generally feel about the person you just lost to? Are you looking forward to spending more time with them?

Anytime we "win" an argument with someone, it automatically means that they "lose."

Allyson—Pushed to Prove Her Point

Allyson loves her job in finance and in fact just got a promotion. Despite her success, she wanted to be seen by her colleagues as smart and deserving of her new role and so felt the need to prove herself every day by telling them when and why she disagreed with them about anything and everything. Arguing her position was about more than being right; it was really about her need to be respected. Her very identity was tied up in scoring those gratifying wins. In the meantime, winning her point felt good in the moment, but when people began to distance themselves from her, the result was the exact opposite of the validation she needed.

*We worked with Allyson on using pauses, listening strategies, and her Parking Lot to stop being so unintentionally combative in her communication, and more importantly on learning to respect—and trust—*herself *and her ability in her new role. Once she started feeling better about herself and more confident, she was less self-conscious, was able to listen more attentively, and could lead without the need to undermine her coworkers just to make herself look "good." Her relationships and career improved immensely, became a lot more enjoyable, and her colleagues began to recognize and appreciate her intelligence when she was no longer using it to assert her right to be a leader.*

People with ADHD tend to be argumentative because arguing is super stimulating, very emotional, we want to be seen as right, and it feels a bit like a game—at least to *us*. For others, talking with someone who's argumentative makes them feel defensive and interrogated. It's a huge turnoff that can cause people to avoid dealing with you at all. It's not effective communication because it is all about winning and being "right" in that moment, not listening or exchanging information, and every win equals a loss for the other person. One way you can defuse your tendency to argue is to turn things around, and instead of trying to prove your opponent wrong, clarify or validate what they're saying to help them feel understood.

You: So, is this what you meant when you said *x, y, z*?

Them: Yes! Of course . . .

You (focused on where they're coming from): Okay, I understand. I see that . . .

It takes (at least) two people to argue, and it's always your choice whether to be one of them.

If it's not a life-or-death discussion, which it usually isn't, you can choose to focus on reaching a more meaningful goal, like maintaining your connection with someone. Or you can simply respectfully disagree with them and move on without needing to win or have them lose. It takes (at least) two people to argue, and it's always your choice whether to be one of them.

☑ Have the Courage to Be Wrong (and Happy)

In any conversation, remember your initial intention for the communication. Then, if you realize that you may in fact be mistaken about something, and you're feeling especially brave, simply (or not so simply) admit that you're wrong as soon as you can.

Truthfully, this is not easy. To admit that we're wrong feels like conceding that everyone in our life was right about *all* the criticisms we've heard (or imagined) about ourselves. We aren't qualified. We aren't smart. We aren't competent. We don't deserve to be where we are. But needing to be right has never made people love (or respect) *anyone* more. It's the exact opposite. Being trapped by a compulsion to always be right eventually makes the people you love the most dread communicating with you and feel the need to walk on eggshells all the time when talking to you. Which I'm guessing isn't what you ultimately want.

As Dr. Gerald G. Jampolsky wrote: "You can be right, or you can be happy." A lot of us are so busy trying to prove ourselves right and others wrong that we've lost too many amazing, well-meaning friends, deep relationships, and supporters along the way.

People with ADHD tend to struggle with communication; however, by increasing your focus and intention, improving your listening skills, avoiding arguments, pausing, and being prepared to handle the impulsive need to blurt something out, you can absolutely learn to communicate more effectively. This will lead to fewer misunderstandings and genuinely deeper connections with others—something that most of us have always wanted.

ADHD-Friendly Quick Summary

- Communication is the primary way we connect with other people, develop relationships, and shape how we're perceived in the world.
- Speaking in circles, oversharing, interrupting, overanalyzing what we want to say, having no filter, missing what others are saying, being too intense, being confrontational, and repeating ourselves are common communication challenges for people with ADHD.
- Listening is the most important part of communication, and it's impossible to fully listen while you're talking!
- Set your intention before speaking.
- Remove competing stimuli to more easily connect with and listen to others.

(continued on next page)

(continued from previous page)

- Remember to look up and make eye contact when you're speaking with someone.
- Delay conversations when you're overly emotional by writing down what you want to share so that you won't forget, and to create space to regulate your emotions.
- Engage your brain when you're bored listening: Imagine you'll be tested on it later, and try to find the purpose behind what the other person is saying.
- Ask questions to show interest and verify your understanding.
- It takes (at least) two people to argue. You can opt to not be one of them.
- Admitting when you're wrong will almost always lead to people respecting you more.
- Choose to be happy over needing to be right.

ONE FOCUS

Practice Your Communication

You've just read about many proven and effective communication techniques that have worked incredibly well for women with ADHD.

Choose one and only one of these to implement in your communications for just one week.

- Press Pause on Interrupting
- Set Your Intention
- Get Rid of Competing Stimuli
- Unload Carefully
- Practice Out Loud: Role-Play
- Park It
- Engage Your Brain / Listen Actively

- Avoid Jumping to Conclusions by Asking Clarifying Questions
- Converse Without Being Critical
- Have the Courage to Be Wrong

After implementing just one of these methods for only a week, you'll become more cognizant of your role in your communications and experience how much power you truly have in creating, building, and repairing the relationships in your life!

Now that you are armed with results-based strategies for managing many of the most difficult challenges for women with ADHD—like communication, mood management, time management, making decisions, staying on track, staying organized (you're well on your way to being on top of those things now, right?)—the strategies and concepts coming up in part 4 will allow you to go one step further. Getting things done is great, and that might seem like all you need right now, but it's just the tip of the iceberg. The real end goal is what you will be able to accomplish with the countless new opportunities that open up *as a result* of better managing your ADHD! This is where you get to think bigger, connect to your heart, and look toward what's truly possible.

PART IV

Beyond ADHD Management

Bringing Your Awesomeness to the World!

The insights presented in this section have inspired massive breakthroughs for many thousands of clients over many years because they've allowed them to focus on who they are BEING, versus what they are DOING.

In these next chapters, you'll get to go beyond the practicalities of overcoming specific ADHD challenges and look at the bigger picture that will help you create the life you most want to live. Onward!

23

Connecting with Yourself

Over the years, I've heard an incredible variety of stories from clients, and I can relate, one way or another, to nearly all of them. Despite how different their lives, careers, perspectives, experiences, strengths, and challenges may be, I've learned that many women with ADHD share a similar inner experience.

- We've grown up never quite understanding why we don't seem to fit in and why it feels like no one truly gets us.
- We think incredibly fast, which contributes to a pervasive sense of restlessness. If the rest of the world were as quick as we are, we'd be living in the twenty-third century already. Sometimes we feel like a cheetah living among sloths while paradoxically still feeling that we're behind everyone else!
- We're extremely sensitive, and whatever is happening around us gets absorbed into every aspect of our being. Overall, we experience considerably more overwhelm, emotional upheaval, and more anxiety than neurotypical people.
- We're frequently frustrated with ourselves, dissatisfied with our lives, and dwell on what should be better.
- We often (if not always) feel stressed out and disconnected from ourselves, and struggle to keep our lives from unraveling.

One of the biggest reasons your life can sometimes feel out of control is because of how hard it is to slow down to reflect on anything about yourself while you're running around in constant reaction mode—which is all the time. If your ADHD isn't managed, you could easily spend the rest of your life feeling like a Ping-Pong ball being forcibly bounced from one thing to another.

THE DANGER OF DETACHMENT

When your brain is always a thousand steps *ahead* of you, yet you're still behind on the twenty-five things you should have done yesterday, today's tasks are already slipping away, and you are also chasing down the multiple things you want to do tomorrow, it's not surprising that you're super stressed out with zero time to take a breath, let alone acknowledge and check in with what you are experiencing, feeling, and wanting. It's as if you're ahead of yourself, completely behind, and trapped in one place all at once.

Our brains are juggling so many different things, it can feel like we're always trying to catch up with something, so the idea of connecting to what's important, or having the bandwidth to reflect on where we're going in our lives, seems not only impossible but completely absurd! If we could only connect more deeply to ourselves, we wouldn't be living on the surface of our lives nearly as much—but because our minds move so fast, it's hard to slow down enough to go deeper and develop that connection. It's a classic catch-22. Ultimately, there's a danger of things feeling so out of control that we can start to feel detached or dissociated—from ourselves, the people we love, our goals, and, quite frankly, everything!

How does this happen? How does such an extraordinary, passionate, brilliant, bright-light, high-speed thinker end up feeling completely detached, burned out, and unfulfilled?

The answer is disconnection.

It can feel like you're watching your life through a screen. You're doing the things you normally do, but you're not fully experiencing them because your mind is simultaneously somewhere else. Meanwhile, the inner you craves the depth of more meaningful connection, which you can't achieve while existing on the periphery of your own life. If you sometimes (or always) feel as if life is happening *to* you at high speed, and *often* think, *Wait, did I just do that?* then you know what it means to be disconnected.

One of the massive paradoxes of ADHD is that for someone who feels absolutely *everything* so intensely, after years of living with that constant high volume (in your mind), you can become somewhat desensitized. It's like wearing high-grade earplugs at a concert. You're at a great show and you hear everything, but the music is muffled and doesn't feel as full as it should. There's something between you and the complete experience of the moment. This feeling of detachment and disconnection can go on for years or possibly your entire life.

If you sometimes (or always) feel as if life is happening *to* you at high speed, and *often* think, *Wait, did I just do that?* then you know what it means to be disconnected.

A Disconnected Reality

That's pretty much where I was in my early thirties. I was living on Manhattan's Upper West Side in one-third of a bedroom—my roommate used the other two-thirds of the room as her art studio. It was the least expensive space I could find, and it suited me just fine (except for when my roommate was hit with inspiration to paint at 4:00 a.m., which happened more often than you'd think).

I was working at a nonprofit job, barely getting by, dating a lot, being in my comfort zone of "being busy being busy," and living on the edge of the unknown. Back in those days, for many of my peers, being in our thirties meant we were "supposed to be" in a committed relationship with kids, or at least on a promising career path, or both. Basically, be an adult.

I, on the other hand, was broke, very single, and on a dead-end career path. I felt anxious about my future, and whether I'd ever have a life my parents (and grandparents) would approve of, and although it was "interesting," my life had been feeling two-dimensional for some time. As time went by, the restlessness, pressure, and intense impatience for my "real" life to begin made me feel more agitated and even less in control.

Life was quickly happening to *me on all levels, and drama and chaos became my everyday reality, all in the name of doing everything possible to move toward what I thought I wanted. Over the course of three years, I got married, divorced, engaged to someone else, became single again, and then became involved with a guy who turned out to be prone to addictive and abusive behavior. Ultimately, he was the cause of the absolute worst and most chaotic year of my life. It felt like I woke up one person, and by the next day, my entire existence and self-identity had been turned completely inside out and removed from everything I knew myself to be. The last day of our relationship was that day. The craziness had reached a level that surpassed anything I had ever imagined facing. Working my way through the personal trauma I experienced at that time was an extreme and unwanted stimulus that shook me deeply. Over the next few years I slowly pulled myself back together. But still—no woman should ever be moving through her life so fast, in constant reaction mode, and so oblivious to what's going on around her that she loses all self-awareness and finds herself in horrible (and preventable!) situations. And yet, in different ways, many of us do.*

During those years, my life was feeling like a series of unedited scenes in a very disjointed low-budget movie about a life gone wrong. Everyone around me could clearly see that things were unraveling at breakneck speed and getting completely *out of control, and finally, for the very first time, I saw it, too.*

Then, in the wake of that wreckage, after begrudgingly having to move back home for a few months, I met the doctor who diagnosed me and literally told me I was the "poster child for extreme ADHD." As harsh as that sounds, it was the most positive thing he could have said about me. His diagnosis answered so many questions I had been asking myself for as long as I could remember. It was also possibly the very first time in my life I ever felt remotely understood.

Once I found out and accepted that I have ADHD, I was able to look at myself objectively. I realized that practically everything I had done throughout my life was driven by a need for stimulus and to avoid feelings of stagnancy, no matter what the cost. I was living in constant reaction mode and had created zero space to slow down to connect with what mattered to me.

Having that realization of what I was dealing with was the first time in my life that I felt connected to myself. That connection gave me tremendous power to make different types of choices. Instead of thinking, What kind of adrenaline, fun, or excitement is out there? *my thought process switched to,* If I only have one life, which may very well be the case, what kind of life do I want to create?

Going forward, every decision—which men to date, what jobs to take, where to live—became a question of seeking deeper happiness versus instant stimulus. I was able to get really clear about the relationships I had been in and why I had stuck around for the excitement, confrontations, risk-taking, and everything in between.

The same realization helped with my work situation. I finally saw that I'd been jumping from one job to another, always looking for a new game to play and a new start. It was never boring, but in terms of my career progress, I was completely stuck in one very small, emotionally claustrophobic place. I knew that my ultimate goal was to help people. However, the actual work I was doing didn't allow me to help people directly.

Once I became much better at managing my own ADHD and was able to start helping others with similar challenges, I found that the thrill of moving to different cities for different jobs paled in comparison to the excitement and experience of legitimately helping people one-on-one and sharing in their breakthroughs.

I had another big realization during this time. It finally dawned on me that all those people who were living what I had judged to be unbearably boring lives were genuinely quite happy. Unlike me, they were largely content with the choices they had made. And contentment looked really good. I don't think I had ever experienced that before! I wanted more of what they had, whatever that was.

HOW TO CONNECT WITH YOURSELF

During my quest to learn everything possible about how to manage my own ADHD brain, one of the things I did after receiving my diagnosis (since I was between jobs anyway) was to backpack through India for nine weeks to fully immerse myself in practices that might help me quiet my racing mind and connect more deeply with myself. I even spent a week in Dharamshala trying to meditate in the presence of His Holiness the Dalai Lama (an adventure story for a different time). Despite being in a small group with the Dalai Lama, Buddhist monks, and only a few other travelers, I couldn't sit or calm my mind for even sixty seconds and ultimately failed miserably at meditating.

I did, however, realize something completely different during those weeks in the mountains of India. I found that the way to quiet MY mind was the exact opposite of what everyone else was telling me. Rather than attempting to sit through more meditation sessions, I went for short hikes by myself and discovered that when my heart rate was faster, my mind was calmer, which amplified my ability to go deeper! I *was* able to achieve a sense of connection, quiet, and calm while on a hike—or doing anything that challenged my body in some small way—which allowed me to answer the deeper questions I was asking myself.

That's how the Time-In exercise, a technique that has been extremely impactful for so many, was created. Although moving quickly and responding to questions largely contradicts the idea of finding peace and calm through being still and "quieting your mind," taking a Time-In helped me find a path to inner connectedness that so many women with ADHD crave.

☑ The Mind-Body Time-In

A Time-In is a brief physical activity immediately followed by asking yourself questions while you are still out of breath. In other words, you can begin to connect with yourself and who you are underneath all the chaos by getting out of your head and into your body (remember state changes?). It's best to do this outside if you can.

You can begin to connect with yourself and who you are underneath all the chaos by getting out of your head and into your body.

Start with a quick speed walk until your heart rate is elevated, run in place, or walk up and down the stairs five times—whatever works for you based on your fitness level. My personal go-to with our clients is to take them outside during their coaching session and have them run or move as fast as possible for exactly two minutes. The key here is to reach a point of being slightly out of breath, which will take you out of your head, out of your emotions, and directly into your physical body, where your mood is less likely to influence your answers.

Once you are in your body and a bit winded, focus on one of the questions from the list below. Record a voice memo or scribble out your answer with the very first thoughts that come to mind. These are usually your "best" and most true responses.

Here are some questions that will help you start to connect with yourself:

Time-In Questions

1. **What do I want?** If you don't know, try asking: *What did I once want—even if it was forty years ago?*

2. **What matters to me?**

3. **What (or who) gives me energy?** *When, and with whom, do I feel most invigorated?*

4. **What (or who) drains my energy?**

5. **What am I good at, and how do I know this is true?** If you don't know, try asking: *What have other people said I'm good at?*

6. **What's something I feel proud of?** *What part did I play in making it happen?*

7. **Who do I wish I could be more like?**

8. **What do I want more of?**

9. **What do I want less of?**

Use your answers to these questions as a catalyst to kick-start your journey of reconnecting with yourself and what's important to you. You will likely have to repeat the Time-In exercise several times to really get to your core truth, and by writing out your answers, they'll be available for when you feel like your life is a runaway train, or you feel stressed out or disjointed.

When I came back from India and wanted to continue reconnecting with myself, I'd go outside and speed-walk for about twenty minutes with a tiny pad of paper and a pencil. I'd think about only one or two of the questions each time and wrote down whatever words came to me. Writing on paper versus recording a voice memo also helped to keep my answers brief and closer to the essence of my thoughts. When I got back home, I'd take out the pad of paper and expand on what I had scribbled down on my walk. On a personal note, the last two questions—*What do I want more of?* and *What do I want less of?*—were particularly enlightening for me.

Erika—Work-Life Balance

Erika is a single mom who is trying to balance a very demanding job with raising her eight-year-old daughter. She struggles with a lot of guilt because she feels as if she's always falling short, dropping her kid off late to school almost every day, being late for work, and being distracted by work while she's with her daughter. She feels like she is in a no-win situation. If she prioritizes her job over her child or vice versa, everything in her life will fall apart: either she'll lose her job or she'll let her family down and feel like she's a terrible mother. No matter where she is, she feels she is not giving enough, doing enough, or being enough, and she lives in constant reaction mode.

Like so many women we work with, Erika only sees her failures. If you point out a success, she'll say, "Oh, I was just lucky that worked out," and she habitually thinks that everything she does is wrong or not enough. At her job, no matter what she's doing, Erika interprets her boss's comments as either a criticism or a demand that she must handle immediately, and when she's at home, she constantly thinks her daughter is disappointed in her.

Along with the pervasive sense of failing, Erika feels as if she's missing out on life because she's not present in almost anything she does. Whether it's her job or her family, she never feels like she's really there—or anywhere.

Erika's First Time-In: Choosing More and Choosing Less

When I had Erika do the Time-In exercise, she spent three minutes walking up and down the stairs in her home relatively quickly. I asked her to immediately answer these questions:

What do I want more of? *To feel secure. Trust. I want more time with my daughter.*

What do I want less of? *If there was one major thing in my life I could do without, it would be to stop believing that I'm messing everything up. To stop being so certain that I'm failing my daughter and to not wake up scared every single day thinking "I'm going to get fired today."* (Basically, to let go of her feelings of deep insecurity.)

Erika's answers revealed how she feels and reacts to situations. She spends time with her daughter, but she doesn't feel present or connected during that time because she is always trying to multitask when they are together. To Erika, more time with her daughter means more quality time, or connected time, not simply more minutes.

Erika needed to learn to trust that she had legitimately earned the job and position she holds *before* she could short-circuit the feeling of "everything is about to fall apart." She's not going to lose her job or end up homeless if she puts off responding to an email while she's with her daughter, and when it comes to her job, **as long as it doesn't involve an ambulance or the ER, most emergencies are *perceived*, not *actual* emergencies.**

By using some of the emotional management tools we discussed earlier—like the cost-benefit analysis and Facts Are Friendly, as well as taking the time for her to go deeper with herself and answer her Time-In questions—Erika was able to start seeing that she has many strengths and, for the first time, began to believe and trust that she's gotten to where she is because of what she's done so effectively. Her job and success didn't come to her by magic. She earned them and doesn't need to live her life with an underlying worry that she'll lose everything if she is totally present with her daughter for a few moments!

This Time-In exercise has worked for thousands of women like Erika, regardless of what stage of life they're in.

Jade—Handling High School

Jade is an incredibly bright high school senior who was diagnosed with ADHD when she was seven. When she puts in the effort, she gets straight A's and does brilliant work far above her grade level. The trouble is that most days, she feels irritable, bored, and unmotivated. Not only are her grades slipping, she isn't doing anything to prepare for college. When asked if she cares about her academic future, she says yes, but then she turns around and spends most of her time gaming and texting.

Jade's parents want to do whatever they can to help her succeed, so they take her around to tour colleges (she says they drag her), enroll her in extracurricular activities, and are constantly on her, giving her everything and trying to manage her life for her in a way that (they think) will get her into the best college so she can succeed in life. They don't realize that by jumping in and micromanaging, they're doing more harm than good. What their ADHD daughter really needs is a chance to personally experience and feel for herself what she might want.

Jade's First Time-In

Because Jade often felt unmotivated, we started with a Time-In to assess her gut reaction about what would boost her mood and give her more energy. During our sessions, I had Jade walking as fast as she could through her neighborhood and answering Time-In questions for over a month before she was able to get connected to her inner truth. Eventually she came to these realizations:

What drains my energy? *Gaming all day, spending hours staring at a screen, messing around on social media, and chatting with certain people who leave me feeling tired and annoyed.*

It took Jade by complete surprise (it truly shocked her) to realize that besides boring classes that she didn't like, her energy was depleted by the activities she defaulted to habitually all day.

What gives me energy? *Interesting new topics and challenges to solve.*

When Jade was able to identify the things that drain her and leave her feeling exhausted and cranky and then connect the negative feelings of lethargy with spending time on these activities, she was able to decide **for herself** how to limit the amount of time she devoted to these activities each day. Otherwise, she could have easily spent her entire life feeling unmotivated, resentful of her parents, disappointed in herself, and unfulfilled.

What Jade wanted to do was explore a variety of interests that light her up by trying them, not just hearing or reading about them. The interests don't have to be things she thinks she might be good at or that will make her "successful" by someone else's standards. They have to be things that make her smile and feel fulfilled while she's doing them! By exploring chemistry, creative writing, computer programming, graphic design, and even entrepreneurship, she unlocked a universe of possibilities for herself by getting connected to what genuinely energized her.

When you can reconnect with yourself, truly amazing things happen. One thing that often occurs for our clients is simply getting clear on their true priorities, sometimes for the first time ever. They see what they really need and want to be doing, instead of running around on autopilot reacting to absolutely everything coming at them.

STEPPING OUT OF REACTION MODE

Few women with ADHD have a life others would describe as calm, peaceful, grounded, or quiet. Yet we all need to incorporate at least some calm and reflective time into our lives in order to stay connected with ourselves and maintain some control over the direction we're headed.

You definitely don't need to take a journey to the Himalayas to learn how to ground yourself—unless you want to (it's really beautiful). Beyond the Time-In exercise, you can intentionally press Pause in your day and step out of reaction mode to deepen your connection to yourself on a more regular basis.

☑ Ground Yourself

This is going to sound overly simple, but try it for a few days. Find a calming activity that you enjoy doing, that is not strenuous, and carve out just a few minutes a day to do it. Some examples might be drawing or doodling; journaling or writing; a hands-on activity like cooking, woodworking, gardening, doing your hair and makeup (relaxing for many); going through pictures of yourself from a time when you were feeling strong or powerful; singing or praying. Choose anything that creates a feeling of calm and joy for you.

While you're doing the calming activity, intentionally think about something positive in your life. This could be something you've done that you're proud of or that you're happy to have, or something you love or are looking forward to. You could also ask yourself any of the Time-In questions we talked about a few pages ago. The point is to create a comfortable background "white noise" with your calming activity that helps to quiet the spiraling thoughts in your mind so you can focus on specific thoughts that bring you a tiny bit closer to yourself.

Create a comfortable background "white noise" with your calming activity that helps to quiet the spiraling thoughts in your mind.

BECOMING SELF-AWARE

Hopefully by now you know that you are not your ADHD, and you understand the importance of connecting with yourself, as well as how to start managing many of your most challenging ADHD symptoms. Yet still you may find yourself automatically reacting out of fear, impatience, or frustration, even if you are no longer always living in reaction mode. What's up? Because you have been doing all the things I'm suggesting (right?), shouldn't you be a happy, focused, and empowered picture of serenity by now? The truth is that there is a lot more to you than you may realize. In fact, there might even be more "*yous*" to you than you realize!

WHO'S DRIVING THE BUS

All of us, whether or not we have ADHD, behave differently depending on the role we're playing, the situation we're in, who we're with, and what we're doing. This is an approach designed to help you understand and recognize *allll* the different aspects of your personality so that you will have more power (and perspective) to decide which part of you will be in control.

1. Consider the many different roles you play and the varied aspects of your personality that show up when you're in different situations. There's the supportive friend, the overwhelmed ADHDer, the impulsive ADHDer, the ambitious entrepreneur, the life of the party, the oppositional colleague, the worried mother, the confident leader, the stressed-out leader, the spiritual seeker, the anxious daughter, the procrastinating student, the impatient customer, and so on. You can probably name about twenty

more that you see in yourself. Give all your personas (or as many as possible) a name or a label so that you recognize them more easily going forward.

2. If it's not easy for you to identify the different aspects of your personality, ask yourself these questions about who you are in different situations in your life, and write them in your notebook:
   * Who am I when I'm achieving something I really, really want? (For example, this could be your driven, goal-oriented self.)
   * Who am I when I'm putting off doing something important? (This could be your overwhelmed, fearful self.)
   * Who am I when I'm holding someone I love? (Your nurturing, affectionate, connected self?)
   * Who am I when I'm criticizing and arguing with my partner? (Your defensive, fearful, or confrontational self?)
   * Who am I when I'm out with my best friends? (Your social, relaxed, carefree self?)
   * Who am I when I don't care about anything anymore? (Your apathetic or resigned self?)
   * Who am I when I'm cursing the traffic I'm stuck in? (Your frustrated, stressed-out, or impatient self?)
   * Who am I when I'm failing miserably at something? (Your self-critical or defeated self?)
   * Who am I when I'm worrying incessantly and can't stop? (Your fearful, anxious, insecure self?)
   * Who am I when I'm trying to prove that I'm right? (Your argumentative, insecure, or competitive self?)
   * Who am I when I'm totally focused on something I deeply care about? (Your passionate, hopeful, dedicated self?)

If you're still having a hard time thinking about the different aspects of your personality, it sometimes helps to think about the people who influenced you—even before you were born! Consider your unique background and lineage, your family members, or what you know about the ancestors you never met who survived the most difficult times in history so that you could be here now. Their genes are woven into your DNA! Fact.

Give all your personas (or as many as possible) a name or a label so that you recognize them more easily going forward.

3. Now imagine a big yellow school bus, and on this bus, each seat is occupied by a different aspect of your personality. What a fun bus! In your notebook, write down the names you gave to each of your personas. Feel free to note the specifics about each one—like how they look, dress, or speak differently from the others. If it helps, think of TV or movie characters whose look and personality they might resemble.

4. From this list, identify your three or four most prevalent personas—the ones who show up most often—and write them down.

5. Now think about which of your personas tends to focus on the challenges, negatives, and perceived shortcomings you have in your life, and write those names down. Is there any overlap with these negative personas and your prevalent persona list?

   Do you notice how often you allow these parts of yourself to be in the driver's seat of your life?

6. Next, take one minute to think about the version of yourself or the persona you wish you *could* be most often—at home,

at work, and throughout your life. Maybe you have one or two favorites, and when they're in charge, you happen to feel pretty amazing. Write them down—are they also on your prevalent persona list? If not, a shift in thinking can help move them over to that list.

Focus on these happy, strong, loving, energized, achieving, and positive aspects of your personality and visualize them in the driver's seat of your bus. With them in control, envision how you're approaching the things you need to do, how you're behaving with the people you spend time with, and how you're feeling and living on a day-to-day basis. This version of you is as real and achievable as any image you have of yourself.

It's important to recognize that none of your personas define you—including the ones who are controlled by your ADHD. They are each simply one small aspect of you. When you know which facets of your personality are on your bus, you can recognize your favorite "passengers" and bring them forward to take the wheel whenever you want!

It's important to recognize that none of your personas define you—*including the ones who are controlled by your ADHD*. They are each simply one small aspect of you.

7. When you find yourself feeling or behaving in a way you don't like, think about the bus and who (which part of you) is driving it in that moment. By being aware of who is driving, you can then consciously switch drivers! Just imagine one of your favorite passengers (personas) standing up and moving to the front, taking over the driver's seat, and driving the bus!

The goal of connecting with yourself is to feel whole and grounded—which, for many of us, is a game changer. It will enable you to step outside of perpetual reaction mode, even if it's only for a few minutes a week, and take a break from the continuously noisy, pulled-in-a-million-directions-all-at-once stimulus that you've grown used to. You'll then be able to accomplish what you want more easily by understanding, connecting with, and guiding *all* aspects of the extraordinary person who's reading this sentence—you.

24

Uncover Your Purpose

This chapter is in honor of all the outstanding and inspirational women who have come to me for help over the years and once they became experts at managing their ADHD found an entire new world of opportunities open up for them. Many of those brilliant women have created amazing new realities for themselves and others, from their family lives to their careers, to their personal legacies and more—none of which would have been remotely possible if they had continued living their lives in reaction mode, desperately just trying to be more organized and on time.

I've devoted a lot of the pages in this book to how to do things, but I want you to think more broadly than that. This chapter is not so much about the *how* but the *who,* as in, who are you ***being*** when you live your life, interact with others, and pursue your dreams, and how do you keep moving forward to be your *favorite* version of yourself? It can all start when you begin living purposefully and bringing more meaning into your everyday life. You started this process through discovering your Big Why; now it's time to go bigger.

Living with purpose goes far beyond simply wanting to be on time, be more organized, and feel less stressed out. In essence, having a greater purpose is the biggest, most gigantic Big Why behind what you want—it gives your life meaning! It doesn't mean you have to devote your entire life to world peace or another huge worthy cause. Let's be real—some of us are still trying to figure out why we don't have any clean socks left when it feels like we *just* did our laundry. Either way, for those of us with ADHD, finding ways to bring more meaning into our lives can lead to a less immediate yet massive benefit—it helps to direct your focus on what's important, making it much easier to avoid distractions.

At a certain time in my life, the idea of ever having a greater purpose beyond remembering to feed my dog twice a day was unimaginable. Basic survival felt overwhelming enough; how could I consider something bigger? But after receiving my ADHD diagnosis, I developed techniques to manage my own brain, and friends who saw my life *finally* starting to come together began asking for help.

Discovering My Purpose

I remember exactly when I had a (rare) moment of clarity and decided that my purpose for the next few years was to help as many adults with ADHD as I could—people just like me. I was working at a(nother) nonprofit job and was responsible for creating a health and fitness coaching program for hundreds of government employees. I didn't know very much about health or the technicalities of fitness, but creating the coaching program came naturally to me. In fact, my program was turning out to be more successful than anticipated, and the participants were loving it! During a late-night planning session for the grand finale awards celebration, I realized how much better it would be to develop a coaching program for people I really "get," care about, and feel connected to—people with ADHD who were experiencing similar challenges and pain in their lives to what I had gone through. The idea of helping them filled me up so much it felt uncontainable. Over the past many (many!) years living with that very purpose has continued to motivate me, guide my decisions, and has almost completely taken away my urge to jump ship into a shinier, newer, or more "exciting" career—about 95 percent of the time (just being honest here).

Regardless of how much life experience we've had, it's not always clear what our greater purpose is, and it often feels overwhelming to even think about it. This is when you can narrow your focus and set a purpose for a *part* of your life—as big or small a part as you want. You can choose a purpose for the next few years—or the next few months. Or it can be the purpose you have for your relationships, your career, or a greater purpose for your personal growth . . . really, for any area of your life!

Ella—A Deeper Purpose at Work

Ella is a nurturing mother and loving wife in her mid-fifties. After a tumultuous and traumatic childhood growing up in the foster care system, she took a job at a nonprofit devoted to kids in foster care. She is driven, loves her work, and will do anything for her family, which means that she tends to spread herself a bit thin most days.

What Ella wanted more than anything in her career was to make a difference for foster kids, and although her work was effective for the most part, there was one project she wanted to create that wasn't getting the funding or support it needed.

Soon after we started meeting with Ella, she identified her greater purpose, which was to create a space for the kids in foster care to live when they turn eighteen and age out of the system. We had Ella tap into the emotional impact of the proposed project, imagine what the space would look like, how these young adults would interact in it, and how it would feel for each of them to have a warm, familiar place they could come back to whenever they wanted.

When Ella realigned herself with her greater purpose for these kids, she brought her proposal to the board, and they allowed her to shift her energy and perspective so that almost all her fundraising and grant writing at her job went toward raising money for the space she wanted to create. It took nearly a full two years to raise the money she needed, but connecting to her greater purpose helped Ella remain committed the entire time, ensuring that it happened.

☑ START WHERE YOU ARE

With our help, Ella was quickly able to realign with her greater purpose at work. However, many women with ADHD who have spent years in "survival mode" feel as if it is too late to find that kind of deeper purpose. They have a mortgage to pay, a family to support, and dozens of other obligations or people relying on them. They may think they're too old or tired or that what they wanted is no longer possible.

While most people can't drop everything to suddenly pursue greater meaning in their lives, that doesn't mean that you are fated never to find it—even if you got sidetracked eighty times in the past few decades (or weeks). There's a middle ground where you can work your way back to what you feel pulled toward. You can reconnect with what's most meaningful for you and gradually grow your life in that direction.

To start your journey of infusing more meaning into your life, take out your notebook and spend five minutes writing down your responses to this simple (and yet *not* so simple) question:

What is personally important to me? Or put another way: What am I passionate about?

At any age or stage of life, you can connect to a bigger purpose from anywhere—working in a steady career with a family and kids to support, in your sixth year of undergrad with no degree yet, or semiretired with a decent career behind you. I have an incredibly inspiring eighty-seven-year-old client, Sherry, who's quick-witted and working on her ADHD management. She wants to be able to focus on her most meaningful life purpose *right now*—to have extraordinary relationships with her husband and daughter. That is what is most important to her, and she's actively doing something about it.

☑ Look for Patterns to Discover What's Important to You

Even when you're pulled in a million directions with everything going on in your life, I'll bet there are some things that naturally bring you joy and capture your attention more than others. Keep in mind that you're not looking for a brand-new career or even a new hobby by thinking about this. The goal is simply to help you reconnect with the interests and values that are already a core part of who you are.

- What creative activities do you enjoy (drawing, graphic design, taking pictures, making music, etc.)?
- What activities did you use to enjoy that you haven't done in years but would be able to if you had the time?
- What productive activities do you tend to get lost in for hours on end?
- What would you want to spend your time doing if money were not an issue?
- What accomplishments are you most proud of?
- When you look at your calendar over the past year (if you kept one), was there anything you did that you would love to do much more often?

Also, think about the people in your life who you have a strong connection with. What traits and characteristics do they have in common? Write these down as well. Some of your friends may seem completely opposite from one another, but they're probably also similar in some regards. How so? Sometimes it's easier to see what we value by looking at what our closest friends value.

Finding What's Meaningful

I have a client who is currently an event planner in LA, a career she chose because she's always loved parties. She feels strongly that a great party brings people together and can make a difference in their lives. She thinks about the people who first met their spouse at a party or the lifelong memories that can be created at an amazing event. While many of us are terrified by the idea of putting on a party, she is amazing at it because it has purpose for her and energizes her.

One of my self-admitted workaholic clients thought her primary mission in life was to make so much money that she would never have to rely on anyone else. That was her main purpose until she was forty-one and had her first baby. Now her focus has completely shifted, and her sole, undeniable purpose in life is to be the best mom ever to her child.

A different client got into real estate because she loved having the opportunity to meet a variety of people and was drawn to the nonstop nature of the business, only to discover that she also feels deeply fulfilled by helping people find a home, and she continues to stay in touch with them for years.

You may think you're not passionate about anything, or you may be someone who's passionate about almost everything. Most people are somewhere in between, but it doesn't matter where you fall on the passion spectrum! Finding what's truly meaningful for you can be as simple as noticing what fully engages your heart. It should be something productive that you *want* to do and that you can dig into and focus on intently. Don't worry if you feel you don't have a ton of raw talent for that pursuit. Trust me when I say to go for it anyway. I've often noticed, and you probably have, too, that the people with a lot of passion, even if they may be lacking aptitude, seem to be much happier than those with lots of talent but very little passion.

Hannah—Building Community

Hannah is a passionate free spirit ADHDer who lives her life immersed in art and music. She's part of the LGBTQ+ community and is a die-hard festival fan, actively participating in ten festivals every year, earning money by selling her art, and she's spent each summer of her life from the age of eighteen achieving her annual goal of attending Burning Man. Going to this massive outdoor festival in Nevada is her passion, and she would have honestly braved a life-threatening sandstorm to make sure she got there every year.

Hannah came to us in her mid-thirties, expressing that she had been feeling unusually distracted for months and having a hard time expressing her creativity in a way that was still meaningful for her. Eventually, after going through processes to help her pinpoint what was important to her, she realized that there was a need for a festival like the ones she had been attending, designed exclusively for her LGBTQ+ community. She wanted to establish an inclusive three-day wellness festival that allowed the people in her community to learn, connect, and nurture themselves in ways that align with who they are. She saw a massive need for this and believed that with her experience, she was the one who had to do it. It was an enormous undertaking, yet her conviction was solid, fueled by years of passion and personal meaning.

You can imagine the logistics involved in putting on an outdoor festival, how many people she needed to enroll to help her make it happen, and how many things can (and did) go wrong with organizing permits, staffing, volunteers, ticketing, security, hiring practitioners for the workshops, entertainment, pre-festival setup, building outdoor showers(!), post-festival cleanup—you name it. Juggling all this is an absolute nightmare for anyone, let alone an ADHDer, and an infinite number of issues to manage could have easily derailed Hannah! Yet absolutely nothing did. Hannah's purpose was so powerfully front and center that, in every situation, every decision automatically came from a place of "Will this help my festival (her purpose) or not?"

Hannah's connection to her greater purpose drove the level of commitment she needed that made the festival a huge success each year. It took her some time to realize where her passion and purpose would lead her, but when she found it, she brought something new into the world that had huge resonance for her. Sometimes our path isn't clear, but when you take the time to consider what already lights you up or where you already love spending your time, you can find your way.

When you tap into your passions and purpose, whether it's something massive, like creating and running an entire outdoor festival, or something more relatable (and also huge), like setting aside fifteen minutes every day of uninterrupted time to do something that's important to you, you can create greater meaning and fulfillment in your life, which will naturally motivate you to continue doing it. However, even when you become great at mastering your ADHD symptoms, your internal motivation to do what's meaningful for you can *still* fluctuate with your moods, and you might need an extra push to stay in the game and connected to your purpose.

STAYING MOTIVATED THROUGH MEANING

Motivation is fascinating. People can spend years dreaming about what they most want for themselves without ever getting off the couch to do anything about it. But as soon as they start to feel bored, anxious, or simply hungry, they'll jump up to resolve those feelings. Although it's well known that avoiding feelings of pain or discomfort is a powerful motivator, the other and much more enjoyable side of the coin is gaining pleasure! ADHDers are naturally motivated to engage in the fun, meaningful, or instant gratification activities that already spark our interest, that we love doing, or that we're compelled to do for a greater purpose!

Writing This Book

Writing this book was incredibly challenging. I know the material inside out and could easily talk about any one of the topics found here (and many more) for days. But I'm not a writer, and organizing, deciding what to include and what to leave out, and trying to keep it structured were nearly impossible for me—especially when the topics are all so interconnected and overlap with each other in every possible way. It's just not how my ADHD brain works. But I have a gigantic purpose in writing this, and I really meant it when I said that my purpose is to help as many women with ADHD as possible. I'm sincerely hoping that this book can help the women I am not able to connect with personally.

Living from that purpose drives me and keeps me motivated not to quit this entire project, even though I've wanted to a hundred times. I keep a picture in my mind of a woman who's a lot like me (maybe it's you?), and she's on her couch reading this and learning at least one new thing that will truly impact her and make a difference in her life! Which means everything to me.

☑ Happy One-Hundredth Birthday!

If you were looking back at your entire life, what would you want your legacy to be? Imagine you're at your one-hundredth birthday party, and there are people standing up to toast you and your life accomplishments. What would you want people to say about you?

With this in mind, see if you can create two or three meaningful intentions for your life and write them in your notebook. Here are two questions to help guide you to some answers:

- What can you imagine yourself being most proud of in your life?
- What are your core values, and how do you express them? For example: love, contributing to society, creative expression (art,

music, writing), family, mentorship, traditions, acts of kindness that inspire others, and so on.

What is something so small—that wouldn't take more than five minutes—that you can do today, or this week, to move yourself a tiny bit closer to that kind of a legacy? Can you do it right now? Hopefully yes, but if not, find a time when you know you can, put it in your (sacred) calendar, and commit to it.

☑ Go for the Win(s)!

There aren't too many things that are more motivating than winning at something that's important to you. Imagine that instead of watching that runner from chapter 20 going to different stadiums and snack bars, it's *you* who's running in a big race! Now, imagine that you are halfway through the race and, although it's close, you take the lead! In the distance, you can see the finish line! You can hear the other runners nearby, but they are all behind you, and there's no doubt that you're ahead and likely to win! Then you see an adorable puppy on the grass next to the track—and you LOVE puppies!

How likely are you to leave the race to run off the track to go play with the puppy? Most of us would be able to ignore the puppy (okay, maybe after a super-quick glance) if we're already in the lead and about to win, no matter how distracted we can get!

When you're on a path that's purposeful for you and you're on a winning streak, it's almost impossible to lose your motivation.

If you ever want to increase your motivation, even if you feel like you may be losing at what you're doing, do your best to set yourself up to be in a WINNING zone. Break down your actions and tasks into the tiniest steps that you are 100 percent certain you can complete (you've done this a few times already, so you're almost a pro by now). Each little step becomes a victory. Then move on to the next small win and the one after that. Almost everyone loves the feeling of winning, especially when you continue to win over and over (at each very small step). When you're on a path that's purposeful for you and you're on a winning streak, it's almost impossible to lose your motivation or succumb to distractions.

By bringing more meaning into your life, you automatically provide your brain with much of what it needs to stay focused and motivated. Plus, as an added bonus, this paves the way for you to create a much happier, more fulfilling, and less chaotic life.

25

Trust Yourself

Warning! This chapter contains information about a major challenge you may not know you have but that affects your entire life! Virtually *all* our clients face this challenge, yet very few are aware of it or its impact until we bring it to their attention. I would go so far as to say it is an issue that affects almost everyone with ADHD—including you—touching every part of our lives because it's fundamental to self-esteem and overall confidence. The underlying challenge?

You don't trust yourself.

Many women with ADHD believe one of our greatest difficulties is that other people don't trust *us*. Which makes sense because it's common for us to be late (a lot), forget (a lot), say things without thinking (a lot), and unintentionally let people down (a lot). And we may have some work to do to regain that trust. Yet for most of us, I can say with total certainty that not trusting *ourselves* is a much bigger issue. I can also say with confidence that working through self-trust issues is one of the deepest levels of adult ADHD management.

Almost every ADHDer I've ever worked with eventually admits that they fundamentally don't believe that they'll do what they say (to themselves) or have confidence in their own intentions. For twenty, thirty, forty years or more, they have let themselves down repeatedly. Now, even when they really *do* mean what they say, somewhere in the back of their minds, there's a voice telling them, with total certainty, that it probably won't happen. Add your additional experience of being misunderstood too often and you have a perfect recipe for low self-trust, low self-esteem, and low self-confidence that influences nearly everything you do as well as how you feel about yourself.

Working through self-trust issues is one of the deepest levels of adult ADHD management.

Even those ADHDers who are high achievers and appear to have it all together may not be aware that a lack of self-trust permeates their lives, but believe me, it's there. Here are a few clues that may reveal its presence:

- ***Decision-making ability*:** You simply don't trust yourself to make good decisions.

- ***Perfectionism*:** Perfectionism is an excellent Band-Aid to overcompensate for a lack of self-trust. For those who feel "I'm not enough, but if I do everything perfectly, I will be okay and *feel* good enough." Perfectionism also feels like safety and helps you believe you can control something (by being meticulous) when it feels like you have no control.

- ***Being hard on yourself while also being an exceptionally high achiever*:** Results are measurable and hard to negate, so you push yourself from one accomplishment to the next, and your achievements become your identity. You believe you are only as good as your latest accomplishment, accolade, or reward.

- ***Constant need for external validation*:** You require validation from the people in your life, your bank account, your wardrobe, your home, the parties you go to, the number of followers you have on social media, and any other way someone else can essentially tell you that you're okay.

Regardless of how lack of trust shows up for you or how often you've let yourself down, you must trust yourself in order to regain (or gain for the very first time) control of your life. Otherwise, everything you already know, including what you've just learned in these pages about how to manage your life with ADHD and achieve what you want, will be sitting in your beautiful mind with nowhere to go. You *need* to trust yourself enough to take the steps to implement whatever you need to do differently. It takes effort and courage, but I see women do this every single day, and you'll be able to get there as well. I promise.

SELF-TRUST STARTS WITH ACCEPTANCE

You can't think about what you really want when you feel terrible about yourself! Building self-trust requires dealing with any disappointment that you feel in yourself. You have to gently confront what you've lost because of what you haven't done in your life (yet), and any pain that you're living with as a result of past mistakes or missed opportunities that arose from living your life trapped in a system that wasn't built for your brain. I mean, how many mistakes do you think a neurotypical person would make trying to be you?

The first step is to accept and forgive yourself.

This is not so simple. But until you let go of the past, regardless of how amazing your ADHD management systems are, it will be much more difficult to make the deeper changes you want. You have to learn to accept what is, what isn't, what was, what wasn't, and what can and will be for yourself. It's only when you achieve self-acceptance that you can move toward trusting yourself more, and create something better.

Audrey—Identifying Her Successes

Audrey was thirty and didn't have a clue about what she wanted to do with her life. She dropped out of three different schools, was unable to finish her degree, and had been fired from her last two jobs. At the time we started working together, she was living in her mother's basement, trying to hold on to another job, blaming herself for all her failures, and becoming increasingly depressed. She saw herself lagging behind all the friends she had grown up with and was convinced she would never amount to anything—ever.

The one bright spot in Audrey's life was improv comedy. Back in high school, she had formed a troupe with two friends, and they continued to perform for free at a tiny local venue every week. Her whole demeanor changed when she talked about her latest show—she spoke much more animatedly and could go on about the gig for a full hour if I let her. It was clear that this was what lit her up, so I encouraged and helped her to prioritize it.

Over the months that followed, Audrey got her troupe together more often. They started getting their very first paid gigs, and although the practices took up a lot of time and the shows didn't pay well, Audrey was thriving. She's very funny and amazing at connecting with her audience! The more she performed improv, the better she felt about herself, which eventually put her in a better state of mind to figure out what the next steps in her life could be.

During one of our sessions, she mentioned that her mom worked as a receptionist at a private school where unique enrichment activities were one of the central features. You can probably guess where we went from there. With some coaching on how to manage her time, plus some ADHD-friendly goal setting, Audrey was able to put together a simple proposal for a "Comedy Improv with Audrey" enrichment class to offer the school. However, even after doing all this, she was convinced that no one would sign up, and if anyone ever did, that the class would fail because she still had an underlying belief that failure was what she did best. Because Audrey thought of herself as incapable, not very smart, and, at the end of the day, unworthy, the proposal ended up just sitting on her bookshelf.

For Audrey to build up enough self-trust and courage to take the next step, we dug around for a few weeks to find her successes, and to her surprise, there were a few, most of which she had totally forgotten. One of the biggest was her success at being an extraordinary big sister to her little brother. She had never thought of this as an achievement, but her brother, who was now twenty-six, adored her and would do anything for her because of her unconditional love for him and her ability to consistently crack him up with nonstop jokes whenever he felt down. Their relationship was untouchable.

Audrey focused on this connection when she thought of how she could impact other kids and eventually was able to trust herself enough to be able to pitch her idea to the school. The school administrators loved it, and the kids who participated in her program loved it—and her—even more. The program filled up in no time. Soon, other schools in the city had heard about her comedy program, and within a year, she was teaching at five different schools each week. The program grew so fast that Audrey had to hire and train other local improv artists to help teach classes.

It was pretty remarkable to see Audrey's world change 180 degrees in just over a year. She went from feeling very depressed, directionless, and living in her mom's basement to running a rewarding (and fun!) program, earning a living doing something that she absolutely loved, and, most importantly, she started believing in herself and thinking that maybe failure *wasn't* what she did best.

When you believe in yourself enough to put your time into doing what you truly love, it can change your life in countless ways. It might mean building on a previous interest that puts you in a better emotional state and helps you feel more satisfied with your life in general. You usually don't know where an interest, passion, or idea will lead or what other people will think of it. You don't know if you'll be "successful" by any traditional measure or even if you'll want to keep doing it forever, and it doesn't matter! As Audrey found out, once she was able to trust and believe in herself again, she was able to take the steps she needed, and her life completely changed.

LEARNING TO TRUST AND BELIEVE IN YOURSELF

Most of us doubt that we can achieve big things, and when we do (and many of us do) we doubt we can hold on to them, even if we've already done it (and many of us have) multiple times before!

You may have failed at a hundred things and felt upset, frustrated, and impatient, like you're at the end of your rope, unable to see a way forward. And while you may dwell on your failures, you have also succeeded in at least one thing. Or ten. Or a hundred, or more. Yet regardless of how many times you've had a success, did you even notice?

When wins happen (and they do), they instantly vanish from our minds and disappear into oblivion, while we hold on tightly to everything else, *especially* what we're not winning at.

So often, we ADHDers are flying at full speed from one reaction to the next that when we do something well, or someone acknowledges us or thanks us, or we help someone else do something great, we barely realize it. We focus on our failures much more than our successes and regard our failures as our truth. When wins happen (and they do), they instantly vanish from our minds and disappear into oblivion, while we hold on tightly to everything else, *especially* what we're not winning at.

☑ Rewrite Your Story

To move toward more self-trust and more confidence, you need to begin by disproving your old story—the one you tell yourself every day—and start writing a completely new story built upon a more objective body of evidence.

We start this process with Facts Are Friendly. Because our stimulus-seeking brains tend to focus on what has gone wrong, taking the time to consider what you have truly (factually!) accomplished will reinforce that you can be trusted to be able to move forward in your life. These facts are the solid and indisputable foundation you can build your new story on.

Start writing a completely new story built upon a more objective body of evidence.

First, take out a piece of paper and write down your most recent successes in the following three categories (when you are done, you can put it on your Wall of Attention to keep your successes front and center):

***Personal life*:** This could be something like getting back into a long-lost pastime, remembering to eat lunch, being on time for something important, nailing a new recipe, getting more sleep, or it could be as monumental as buying a house, staying sober, being able to retire, or completing a marathon.

***Professional life*:** Keeping your desk organized, doing your job well, getting a better job, knocking a presentation out of the park, getting a promotion, taking a small step toward starting the side hustle you've been thinking about for a decade, getting your degree, reducing your workaholic tendencies by starting to delegate tasks to others, getting to work on time for a full week—it all counts.

***Relationships*:** Did you have a good weekend with your family? Get together with someone you haven't seen in a while? Did you manage to *not* fight with your teenager this week? Did you manage *not* to fight with your parents this week? Did you decide to go out on that second date? Was it fun? Did you call your elderly relative back just to check in? Were you there for a friend who needed support?

Next, how did the successes or good things that happened this week, big or small, come about? **What part did *you* play?** Sometimes it's hard to remember our own positive impact, which is why it is important to take the time to write it out. You then have a visual reminder of your successes.

Take a few minutes to write your new narrative in your notebook based on this brand-new (and improved!) factual evidence.

The part that you played in (*big or small success*) was (*what you did*).
I accomplished ______, and I did it by ______.
I managed to ______. Here's what I did ______.

Keep going for a few more minutes and really internalize and appreciate these wins and, more importantly, *how* you accomplished them.

Remember, when something in your life turns out well, it didn't just "happen"; *you* played an important part. So, the next time you think to yourself, *Wow, I can't believe it worked!*, know that it likely happened because of *you*. Feel free to change the *it* to *I* when you think about these events:

It worked = I worked.
It happened = I made that happen.
It's done = I did it.

You did it. And you can do it again. Own it!

The next time you think to yourself, *Wow, I can't believe it worked!*, know that it likely happened because of *you*. Feel free to change the *it* to *I*.

While you can make a Facts Are Friendly list and a story of your accomplishments to put on your wall, you can also get much more creative—something that a lot of my clients love doing! For example, you can make a short presentation on the arc of your career, your current relationship, your parenting journey, or any path you've been on. You can even include personal photos or images. Write a story or make a video about your accomplishments and imagine that you're presenting it to your boss, an investor, or someone whose opinion means something to you. Then actually present it to someone at home if you want. Have fun with it!

☑ Who You Are Being

When you look closely at how you have accomplished something, consider what it says about where you started and where you are now. Think about your accomplishments over the past few months, especially the tiny ones, and write them down. Then, after each one, write an *I* statement about who you were being and which of your personas was in the driver's seat at that time.

For example:

Paid the monthly bills. = I am responsible.

Organized a night out with friends. = I get stuff done. I can be fun! I can take charge.

Made it to a meeting on time. = I am punctual (and organized).

Completed a project for a client (and they loved it). = I am accomplished and good at my job.

Finished cleaning the basement. = I follow through. I'm reliable and keep my word.

Helped someone this week (even if it's someone you didn't know). = I am a helper. I'm a kind person.

Studied for a full two hours last night. = I am focused on my grades. I'm disciplined and committed.

Supportive and available to my friends and family. = I truly care about others.

Continue adding to your list and do your best to internalize every single *I* statement as you write it down. If you're resisting this exercise because you think those things are too small, or "don't really matter," you probably need to do it more often and with more intent. The next step is to force yourself to write these *I* statements more slowly by writing them out with your non-dominant hand.

By teaching your brain to emphasize what you have accomplished, you are starting to rewrite your narrative. Regardless of whether your accomplishments have been small or large—the important point is that you set small, easily winnable intentions, and then you do them again and again. Eventually, your brain will believe that when you say something, you will actually do it. And therefore, yes, you *can* trust yourself.

26

You Can Change

This chapter isn't related to ADHD management specifically; however, it has to do with how we can and do change as people. Which is important and relevant for all of us.

You've probably heard that people don't change. The truth is, I know that they absolutely do, based on what I've seen over and over again with our clients for the past twenty-plus years. *Nothing* in nature stays the same from one year to the next, and neither do you! So, while your innate personality doesn't tend to change much throughout your life, with some effort, your actions, behaviors, how you feel about yourself, and how you approach situations can and do change. And those changes can have a *massive* impact on your entire life trajectory.

***Nothing* in nature stays the same from one year to the next, and neither do you!**

EVERY SINGLE MOMENT IS A NEW BEGINNING

The first time that I realized change was possible for me, I was falling through twelve thousand feet of thin air with my brain screaming, "How was this a good idea?! Of all the stupid things you've ever done, this is by far the most insane!"

For many years, I had thought about skydiving. In my mind, it was the greatest representation of fearlessness and an experience where overwhelm wouldn't find me. I wanted to go all in, which, to me, meant jumping solo (rather than being attached to an instructor in a tandem jump). So I traveled to Alberta, which was the only place in Canada that allowed solo jumps for first-time skydivers, and that's how I found myself with three friends in a tiny plane flying over the Rocky Mountains. I'd been waiting for this moment for years, and I closed my eyes to try to stay calm and be fully present with it.

Then the plane door opened.

It was thunderously loud as a giant wind rushed into the cabin, so strong it felt like my skin would blow right off my face. I looked around, wondering who would be brave (or crazy) enough to go first and saw our instructor motioning to me! Oh crap. *That's right. Yesterday I had volunteered to go first when we were all back in that room, on the ground, right after we spent eight hours training and preparing for the skydive. But come on—that was a lifetime ago!*

No. I shook my head. The whole thing was starting to unravel. It didn't make any sense that the airplane door was wide open while we were this high up in the sky. It was completely illogical that anyone would willingly throw themselves out that door into the open air. And honestly, how incomprehensible of him to expect me to go first.

Every cell in my body knew this was the absolute worst idea ever. But at the same time, everyone was looking at me. I had been so brave yesterday in the comfortable carpeted practice room, but that wasn't really me . . . the real me was here, now, paralyzed, and frozen with overwhelm. Of course, my brain (the one that got me into this mess in the first place) did what it always does in those moments where something has to happen "now"—it stimulated me into action.

Feeling as though I had stepped outside reality, I stood up and made my way to the door. I looked at the instructor and wanted to cry. In response, he held up his hand for a high five. Seriously?! His huge smile followed me as I stepped out of the deafening airplane all alone and onto the ledge.

I looked down. Bad idea.

I clutched the bar at the side of the plane and looked back up to see the instructor watching from the open doorway, waiting for me to let go so he could start getting the other jumpers ready. As I stared into his encouraging eyes, something happened in my head. It occurred to me that this crazy situation, and everything *that could happen in the next few seconds, had completely been my choice. I planned for it. Paid for it. I drove for three days from Toronto to Alberta with my friends. I made it through the training. I got on the plane. I was now standing on the ledge, all because of my own choices. If I chose to go through with this, and if I* stayed alive, *what wouldn't I be able to do? I was a capable person in a world where I could make my own choices. I was free.*

"Okay!" I shouted, loud enough to hear myself. "I'm letting go!"

Maybe not.

Take two: "Okay!" I shouted even louder. "I'm really letting go!" And I did. I fell very, very fast, while the mountains seemed to rush up around me and nothing but rushing air surrounded my entire body. I remember only two coherent thoughts from that moment:

Thought #1: I don't remember what I'm supposed to do if my chute malfunctions. It better open.

Thought #2: I wish I had an instructor with me.

After what felt like an eternity, my parachute opened, slowing my fall to a gentle drift. In that moment, everything became completely quiet. And in that stillness, one thought, which I will never forget, rose into my consciousness.

"Every single moment of existence is a brand-new beginning for absolutely any possibility to occur."

Every single moment. This one. And this one. And now this one. As each moment brought me a little closer on my journey back to earth, all I could think of was that I could choose to make anything happen. And that's a good thing.

Every single moment of existence is a brand-new beginning for absolutely any possibility to occur.

This realization probably seems obvious, but for me, it was an epiphany. When I connect to that thought now, it still feels as amazing and true as when it first came to me. We can (and do) make choices at every moment. And once we make a choice, a thousand new possibilities open up. The possibilities never end. They keep going. Forever.

This means you're *always* free. Even when you feel completely and entirely stuck, you're not. Where you live, what you do for a living, how much money you think you need to feel comfortable, how you raise your children, how you manage your ADHD . . . there are so many things you can change about your life, simply by doing something differently today from how you did it yesterday.

NEW WAY OF DOING = NEW WAY OF BEING

Think, for a second, about how much you've changed since you were small. You look different, there are different people in your life, you have different interests, and so on. For better or for worse, you have already changed, and for better or for worse, you'll continue to do so. The big question is, how?

The first step to conscious change is knowing that you have the power and the ability to decide what change you want. Give yourself permission to go ahead and choose one thing you want to change for now. First, say it out loud, and then write it down in your journal. Now determine the tiniest step you can *realistically* take toward it in the next hour and do it!

Once you start moving forward with small successes, momentum will become your best friend and possibilities will begin to open up for you faster and faster—kind of like compound interest. That's where the *real* stimulus is.

It's Not Easy, but You're Never Alone

Even with all the best ADHD management, self-trust, motivation tools, and systems in the universe, not everything will go perfectly. It never has, and it's not supposed to. When (not if) you feel completely frozen in overwhelm, always know that you're never completely alone even when it feels like you are. There's a giant community of women in the background of these pages, and none of them achieved what they did completely by themselves. Find someone who understands you and/or is willing to support you when it feels like your ADHD is kicking your butt. Maybe it's your spouse or partner, or someone else in your network of friends, family, or groups. You might even give them this book to read to help them understand you better and support you in staying on track. Very few people get from point A to point B on their own (even if they say they did), and it's the same for you. Honestly, sometimes the best support is having an intelligent, trustworthy person to throw you a rope and pull you out from where you're stuck. Reach for it!

You might also want to seek professional help. There are a lot of options out there, but as you know, in the age of infinite, unmonitored websites where anyone can make all sorts of unfounded claims, and we're constantly exposed to people with huge social platforms but not much true value to offer, there is also a lot of misinformation. It's tricky, so make sure you do your research and find someone who is a true expert in adult ADHD management and who has a verifiable track record of success. The doctor or professional who diagnosed you may be a good place to start.

By the way, if you are reading this book because you are the support person for someone you care about who is struggling with ADHD, you are doing something amazing for them, and you just might be the only person in their life who understands them. Thank you!

Living with ADHD and learning to manage it isn't ever easy, but it *is* absolutely doable! Behind every woman I know who has successfully managed her ADHD, there's been a tremendous amount of effort, a lot of tears, a hunger to grow and move forward, and a deep refusal to stay stuck. I've shared in and seen astounding transformations happen for so many people, and this makes it easier for me to see what is possible for you and for us all in the future.

Honestly, no matter how much you might doubt yourself on certain days, if all those women could do it and I could do it, I absolutely promise you that you can, too.

Conclusion

Keep Going (Yes, You Are Truly Limitless)

There is nothing I want more than for this book to make a difference in your life. It doesn't matter if it's a tiny, medium-size, or monumental difference. All that matters is that it makes something feel better for you than it did before.

If out of all the tips and tools in this book, there is only one that you think fits your situation and works for you, that's great. One is all you need for today. Getting started is getting unstuck. When you are moving forward, even the tiniest bit, you are no longer where you were before. You're in a new place, where new possibilities exist.

So, before you close this book, please remember this: You can *know* dozens, even hundreds of fabulous ADHD management tools. But nothing will ever change for you until you start to *use* them. Catch yourself when you find yourself thinking, *Oh, I already know that.* Those words keep the most brilliant people trapped inside their minds. You'll never know how helpful something can be until you've put it into practice for yourself.

Getting started is getting unstuck. When you are moving forward, even the tiniest bit, you are no longer where you were before. You're in a new place, where new possibilities exist.

BUCKLE UP!

Although we've never met, I know you can get unstuck—just please remember to be patient with yourself. Even for a lightning-fast thinker like you, changing the way you do things takes time. It's not all going to happen yesterday, as much as you might need or want it to. Give yourself at least three months of implementing new tools to start to see noticeable changes. Remember, you've been living with ADHD since the day you were born, even if you didn't know it!

Put a note in your calendar for a month from today's date telling yourself, "It's only been one month." It's helpful to do this because you know as well as I do that a month from today, it will feel like an *eternity* has gone by and you may want to give up if your entire life hasn't dramatically changed by then. Pointing out that it has only been four short weeks will remind you that this journey has just started. You can put notes at the two-month and three-month points also. Fortunately, minor changes *will* happen immediately! Write down each success (like reaching the end of this book!) to show yourself how quickly you're actually moving forward.

Minor changes *will* happen immediately!

You've spent most of your life in survival mode, and now it's time for you to shift into a more grounded, thriving mode. Celebrate and build on the successes you've accomplished and think about how far you can still go.

You know what's possible, so trust yourself, buckle up, and enjoy the ride. You and your brain are absolutely magnificent!

Acknowledgments

There are many people who helped me with this book, but first and foremost, I want to thank my family for putting up with me every day throughout this process.

To my one-in-a-googol husband, Jeremy—beyond being my life partner in all things awesome, business partner, proofreader, anchor, and personal double-strength Bubble Wrap, this book would never in a million years have been written without him.

Also, to our daughter, Arielle, for offering such great editing and design advice—even while sneaking everything off-limits whenever humanly possible when I was buried in this book, and to our son, Izach, for "helping me emotionally" (his words) this entire time with my writing—he really did.

I'll always love the three of you past every solar eclipse!

- Thank you also to my always-up-for-everything mom, who was my first unofficial ADHD coach—even when neither of us knew that I (or she) had ADHD—and to my ever-patient dad, who, beyond tolerating most of my shenanigans, also gave me the poster with the two monkeys that said, *"I never make the same mistake twice. Every day I make new ones."* I'm pretty sure growing up seeing those words every day influenced the work I do—in a good way. I think.
- To my uncle Harv, who, from day one, has personally modeled the extraordinary power of mindset—generating positivity no matter how painful or frustrating the challenge. He's truly a marvel, and I'm thankful for the chance to pay his guidance forward in some small way, even as one of his more challenging students.

- And, to the memory of my grandmothers: my nonstop always "busy being busy" bubbie Ray, and to my bubbie Sara, who survived six different concentration camps yet remained the brightest example of pure love, exuberance, hope, and never ever giving up when life feels completely impossible. I'm incredibly grateful for them, their wisdom, and their abundance of love that's still pouring into this world, including with what's in this book.

Another huge thank you goes to those who played a crucial role in the shaping and production of the book itself.

- To Pam Krauss, for envisioning this book in the first place, seeking me out, and inviting me to write it for Macmillan/ Flatiron—despite knowing I wasn't a writer, and that she'd be editing the early (and messiest) versions.
- To the entire team at Flatiron, especially Lee Oglesby, Molly Bloom, Brittany Leddy, and everyone in production, sales, and distribution—for working behind the scenes to bring this book to life instead of it staying trapped inside my laptop forever.
- To Sheila Oakes, because untangling the thoughts in my always-overwhelmed mind—where a million pieces of information feel equally important all at once—was no easy task! Yet she did this while bringing the priceless gift of calm to the most important parts of this writing journey.
- To my outstanding agent Stephanie Tade for her help, encouragement, patience, and for leading me through this publishing adventure with a very much needed Zen-like presence.

Next, I'm immensely thankful for those who work with me every single day, to help adults with ADHD across the world transform their lives in the most profound ways.

- To my kick-butt rockstar team of Expert ADHD coaches—especially those who have been with me for so many years.

There is absolutely no way we could achieve the life-changing results we do for ADHDers without them! I can't imagine any group program, seminar, or podcast led by anyone, anywhere, that comes remotely close to the magic that each of my coaches brings to every single one of our clients with how beautifully and brilliantly they deliver our program. I am so appreciative of their role in our clients' successes, for helping me to narrow down which of our specific coaching techniques and stories to include in this book, for embracing my very unstructured leadership style, and for being such an integral part of my extended family.

- To my remarkable assistant, Breanne Alshin. Can you imagine supporting hundreds of people every day—all with ADHD—who urgently need your response last week even though they literally just reached out ten seconds ago? I'm beyond grateful for her unrelenting commitment and love for our never-ever-easy, yet totally incredible clients as well as her superhuman ability to handle so many things—including the 1001 things we never (ever!) imagined we'd need when we first hired her.
- To all of our clients, past and present: They are the ones who have undeniably proven that what's written in this book works for ADHDers in the real world, year after year after year. I'm truly grateful to all of them for trusting the process and being both feet in their coaching program, even when it's hard—and especially when they really don't *feeel* like it! I hope they always know and remember that everything they accomplish each day is still, always, just the very beginning of what's next!

And finally, to you—for being here, picking up this book, and reading some or all of it. I'm so happy you did, and it means more to me than I can ever say.

Thank you.

Notes

1. Jeffery N. Epstein and Richard E. A. Loren, "Changes in the Definition of ADHD in DSM-5: Subtle but Important," *Neuropsychiatry (London)* 3, no. 5 (2013): 455–58, https://www.ncbi.nlm.nih.gov/pmc/articles/PMC3955126.
2. "Attention-Deficit/Hyperactivity Disorder (ADHD)," National Institute of Mental Health, https://www.nimh.nih.gov/health/statistics/attention-deficit-hyperactivity-disorder-adhd#part_2553.
3. Stephanie Watson, "What Is Rejection Sensitive Dysphoria?," WebMD, May 2, 2023, https://www.webmd.com/add-adhd/rejection-sensitive-dysphoria.
4. F. Dorani, D. Bijlenga, A. T. F. Beekman, et al., "Prevalence of Hormone-Related Mood Disorder Symptoms in Women with ADHD," *Journal of Psychiatric Research* 133 (January 2021): 10–15, doi: 10.1016/j.jpsychires.2020.12.005.
5. Anneli Andersson, Miguel Garcia-Argibay, and Alexander Viktorin, et al., "Depression and Anxiety Disorders During the Postpartum Period in Women Diagnosed with Attention Deficit Hyperactivity Disorder," *Journal of Affective Disorders* 325 (2023): 817–23, https://pubmed.ncbi.nlm.nih.gov/36681302/.
6. Russell A. Barkley, *ADHD in Adults: Nature, Diagnosis, Impairments, and Long-Term Outcome* (Ashland, Oregon: Professional Resource Press, 2008).

Index

About the Author

Shanna Pearson is the founder, program creator, and coaching director of Expert ADHD Coaching, which provides one-on-one personalized, action-based ADHD coaching for adults and is the largest ADHD coaching program of its kind in the world. Over the past twenty-six years, she has been privileged to serve tens of thousands of clients and train hundreds of coaches.

Shanna writes from the perspective and knowledge of what actually works in the lives of adults with ADHD, based on deep experience overseeing 450,000 individual coaching sessions and a lifetime of mastering her own severe ADHD. She has also explored many things that don't work to manage ADHD—none of which are in this book. Shanna has leaped from planes, snorkeled in a school of two hundred whale sharks, walked across an entire country (more than one, actually), and presented from many stages. She scuba dives; invents new ways to help people help themselves; practices karate; hikes up mountains; loves amusement parks, her family, and her family's history; is a great mom (according to her kids, most of the time); and wouldn't change a thing. She can be found online at **ADHDcoaching.com** and **ShannaPearson.com.**

For You:

- ☑ If you'd like personal support applying the strategies in this book (and more), visit **ADHDcoaching.com.**
- ☑ For free templates and resources related to this book, visit **ADHDcoaching.com/invisibleadhd.**